The New Nutrition

From Antioxidants to Zucchini

The New Nutrition
From Antioxidants to Zucchini

Felicia Busch

M.P.H., R.D., F.A.D.A

JOHN WILEY & SONS, INC.

New York • Chichester • Weinheim • Brisbane • Singapore • Toronto

Copyright © 2000 by Felicia Busch. All rights reserved

Published by John Wiley & Sons, Inc.
Published simultaneously in Canada

Design and production by Navta Associates, Inc.

This publication is designed to provide accurate and authoritative information in regard to the subject matter covered. It is sold with the understanding that the Publisher is not engaged in rendering professional services. If professional advice or other expert assistance is required, the services of a competent professional person should be sought.

Library of Congress Cataloging-in-Publication Data:

Busch, Felicia.
    The new nutrition : from antioxidants to zucchini / by Felicia Busch.
        p.   cm.
    "Published simultaneously in Canada."
    Includes index.
    ISBN 0-471-34793-0 (pbk. : acid-free paper)
        1. Nutrition.   2. Antioxidants—Health aspects.   I. Title.

RA784.B87 2000
613.2—dc21   99-051841

Printed in the United States of America

10   9   8   7   6   5   4   3   2   1

For my sister Ivy,
who inspires me with her courageous
battle against cancer

Contents

Acknowledgments

Many people were responsible for the completion of this book. I owe them my heartfelt gratitude.

To Jeff Braun, my original editor at Chronimed. Without you, this book would have never happened. You are responsible for its conception and all the excitement and wonder that goes into starting such a project.

To Nancy Claridge Turner, my friend and critical editor. You guided the book through a turbulent adolescence and helped form much of the spirit of this work.

To Jeffrey Golick, my editor at John Wiley. Thank you for guiding the transformation of my ideas into an organized and thoughtful work. You were given this project late and I am still amazed at how much you accomplished in so short a time. Under your care this book grew to a level of maturity I am proud of.

To my friends and colleagues at Felicia Busch & Associates, Inc., who over the years helped refine the material presented here. Special thanks to Julie Mattson Ostrow, M.S., R.D.; Anne Dworak, M.P.H.; Cassie Schmidt, R.D.; Mikki Kainz Poplawski, M.S., R.D.; Paula Nessa, R.D.; Terri Loree, M.S., R.D.; Lisa Lovekin, R.D.; Sarah Becker, R.D.; and Lori Holladay, R.D.

To the countless students and interns who did considerable research online, in libraries, and at grocery and health food stores. And to the agencies that generously shared their students for field experiences, including: Regions Hospital, University of Minnesota Food Science and Nutrition Department, North Dakota State University, and the University of Minnesota Graduate School of Public Health Nutrition. Special thanks to Michelle Brooks and Jennifer Hall.

To my colleagues who have encouraged me and so generously shared their wisdom. This book was critically reviewed by colleagues who are national media spokespersons for the American Dietetic Association. This group of dedicated volunteer nutrition experts from around the country helped me to refine the nutrition facts presented and include: Susan Adams, M.S., R.D.; Tammy Baker, M.S., R.D.; Leslie Bonci, M.P.H., R.D.; Connie Diekman, Med., R.D., F.A.D.A.; Gail Frank, Dr.P.H., R.D.; JoAnn Hattner, M.P.H., R.D., C.S.P.; Janet L. Helm, M.S., R.D.; Edith Howard Hogan, R.D.; Cindy Moore, M.S., R.D.; Jackie A. Newgent, R.D., C.D.N.; Betty Nowlin, M.P.H., R.D.; Diane Quagliani, M.B.A., R.D.; Sheah Rarback, M.S., R.D., F.A.D.A.; Cynthia A. Thomson, Ph.D., R.D.; Elizabeth M. Ward, M.S., R.D.; and Althea Zanecosky, M.S., R.D.

Special thanks to my husband Kevin, for your patience when deadlines were looming and for your willingness to free up time for me to write. To my sons Matthew, Ryan, and Daniel, I owe you much time and attention you missed while I was busy working on the book. Get ready to collect!

Introduction

It's not acceptable anymore to only pursue a "healthful diet." The recent explosion of scientific information related to how we nourish our bodies has forever altered the role of food. The dramatic change in the foods we eat, shop for, and design has created a new cornucopia of choices. Such choices are often more frustrating than freeing. My goal in *The New Nutrition* is to help cut through the clutter and share the most exciting and reputable nutrition information available today. Yes, you need to choose a healthy balance of foods. You may also need to take supplements. This book will show you how to put it all together.

Two years of research went into the recommendations offered here. The expertise of top researchers, specialists, and nutrition scientists is included. You decide which information applies to your particular set of circumstances. Nutrition is the interconnected science of a host of nutrients and other factors that don't neatly fit into separate chapters. Here's how we did it:

Chapter 1 gets personal. Who you are and how you live will impact your nutritional needs. You'll need to dig into your family history to trace your medical roots and learn how your ancestry may impact your health. Quizzes and checklists will help you put into perspective your risk for the common chronic diseases of our day.

Chapters 2 and 3 cover the old and new basics of nutrition. Calories, carbohydrate, protein, fat, fiber, and water will always be essential nutrients. Nutrient thieves that steal precious components from food are exposed. These chapters are right up front on purpose. Food comes first in the pursuit of health; supplements are just that—something to consider after you've done all you can to eat right.

The secrets of eating styles from around the world and across the ages are explored in Chapter 4. You'll find nutrition plans ranging from Ayurvedic to Zen macrobiotic and dietary guidelines from around the globe. These models will help steer you to the right food fit for your unique circumstances and needs.

Chapters 5 through 8 delve into the nitty-gritty facts about vitamins, minerals, alternative supplements, and herbal products. Learn what they can and can't do to improve (or harm) your health. Where possible, specific amounts and formulations are recommended.

The information in Chapter 9 sums up the wealth of information we have on how nutrition causes, treats, or cures a variety of the most common disorders and diseases.

One book can't possibly provide every answer. In fact, not all the right questions have even been asked yet in the field of food and nutrition. The final chapter will help you become a better nutrition consumer—of both products and services. You'll learn how to spot the quacks and ways to identify junk science.

Sprinkled throughout *The New Nutrition* are signposts to guide you. They include:

Nutrition Actions: specific steps you can take to make changes

Go Figure: the math behind nutrition formulas, measurement units, and calculations

Handy Hotlines: where to call for more information or help with particular issues

Link Ups: our recommended web sites for more depth on a topic or to keep abreast of new research

Selected Studies: there was not room to include all the key or important studies on any topic. Some of the most recent research is highlighted for you. Reading any of these studies (online or in the library) will present you with a whole list of related reference articles at the end of each publication for further exploration.

Much nutrition information is confusing and conflicting. I've tried to translate the science of nutrition into easily understandable key concepts and recommendations. Now I see an even greater challenge. Keeping up to date with the explosion of new information and research is a daunting task. Use the Handy Hotlines and Link Ups to keep current and connected.

I hope this book will inspire you to look more carefully at how you eat and to make those small changes that can add up to huge health benefits. When you do that, you'll be taking a giant leap toward optimal health and happiness.

PART I

Understanding the New Nutrition

1

The New Nutrition

You hold the power to shape your own health through the miracle of food. There are amazing substances in food that can increase your lifespan, improve your appearance, or lift your mood. We are at a scientific crossroads in human history. We know more than ever imagined about how food can prevent devastating disease or heal genetically inherited weaknesses. What you eat has the awesome ability to change your destiny. Whether you are 22 or 92, seize your opportunity now.

In a lifetime, you will eat eighty thousand meals or the equivalent of seventy tons of food and drink. The most recent National Health and Nutrition Examination Survey (NHANES) reports that 80 percent of women and 70 percent of men ate less than two-thirds of the Recommended Dietary Allowances (RDAs) for one or more nutrients. At least one-third of the elderly in the United States are nutritionally deficient, and the problem will grow as our population ages.

Why are we eating ourselves into early death and disability? In less than one hundred years we have transformed our society from the farm to the factory, and now we're speeding down the information superhighway from our padded office chairs. These changes have impacted both our food and physical activity habits.

Why don't Americans consume enough nutrients from foods? Most of us:

- don't eat enough calories to get adequate vitamin/mineral intakes
- eat a limited variety of food without enough fruits, vegetables, and grains
- choose too many processed foods
- take incomplete or haphazardly chosen supplements

Food used to be simple. You or your neighbors grew most of it. Labels were not required because it was easy to tell a bushel of corn from a bucket of berries. Food preparation and cooking were done at home. People ate what was in season and stored extra for the winter months.

Today, grocery store shelves are stuffed with packaged, processed extras. You have to search to find foods that used to be staples. Even "fresh" foods like produce are often several weeks old when they reach your local market. We're also depending on others to select and prepare our foods. Fast-food drive-through lanes and restaurant eat-in and take-out service are replacing the family dining table. A 1999 report from the United States Department of Agriculture's (USDA's) Economic Research Service found that meals eaten away from home are much less nutritious than home-prepared foods. Eating out typically means taking in about 25 percent less fiber, calcium, and iron than you'd get from foods prepared at home. That's a lot of missed nutrition when you consider that in the 1990s we ate almost twice as many meals away from home compared to the 1980s.

Most of us can't—or don't want to—go back to the good old days. With today's food choices you can eat better. More important, optimal nutrition can help you feel good, age more gracefully, and live longer.

NUTRITION FOR A BETTER HEALTHSPAN

It's the dawn of a new era in nutrition. New nutrition includes more than just meeting basic calorie, vitamin, and mineral needs. Nutrition today requires an understanding of new food attributes that can prevent or delay the onset of chronic disease. There needs to be a new awareness of claims for food and supplements that often far outpace the scientific research to back them up.

Never before in human history have people been able to live as long as we can. But with these extra years come a greater chance of developing chronic disease. Disabling diseases can keep you from enjoying a longer life or erode the quality of those extra years. About ten years ago a front-page newspaper headline startled many people. It read: Eat Right, Don't Drink, Don't Smoke, Exercise Every Day and You'll Live Six Months Longer. "Why bother!" was a common response. Is maintaining healthful habits worth a lousy six months? Unfortunately, the real conclusion of that story was buried. The research report found that people who have health-ful lifestyles enjoy a tremendously superior quality of life in their last years. Those who drink, smoke, don't exercise, and make poor food choices often spend their final years in misery, hooked up to machines in long-term care facilities unable to care for themselves. Today's technology can keep almost anyone's body alive indefinitely. It's your spirit, zest for life, and ability to function that make the real difference as you age.

The compelling evidence is that what you eat has a direct effect on your health and potential to enjoy life. Take charge of your health now. Whether this is your first look at nutrition or you're already quite knowl-edgeable, plan a strategy that fits your lifestyle on a long-term basis. This book will help you. You'll discover simple ways to make small changes that significantly impact how you look and feel—both now and in the future.

Don't Settle for Being Average

No one likes to think of themselves as average. Indeed, the whole "nutrition revolution" is aimed toward more personalized, customized eating options. Nutrient requirements for the average American may not be optimal for *you*. Many factors affect your health and well-being. Some of those you have control over, like diet and exercise. At the moment, genetic factors such as family history remain outside of your direct control. Amazingly, that may not hold true for the youngest generation of Americans today.

A great place to start, though, is by comparing yourself to both the average and ideal American. In Chapter 4 you will learn about new-age and age-old eating styles that may prove a better match for your unique lifestyle. As you complete this chapter, you will develop a comprehensive picture of your health and potential health risks. Analyzing what you're doing right now will give you a sense of where to make improvements.

Here's the latest data on the "average" U.S. man and woman (aged 25 to 50), compared to today's ideals. Obviously, you can't change your height, but your food intake and exercise output are within your control. Where do you fit?

	Average U.S. Man	Ideal U.S. Man	Me	Ideal U.S. Woman	Average U.S. Woman
Height	5'10"	5'10"	_____	5'4"	5'4"
Weight	175	166	_____	125	142
Average Daily:					
Calories	2,153	2,708	_____	2,094	1,769
Protein	90 g	60 g	_____	46 g	65 g
Carbohydrate	404 g	393 g	_____	304 g	229 g
Fat	83 g	90 g	_____	70 g	64 g
Fiber	19 g	27 g	_____	20 g	13 g
Cholesterol	203 mg	< 300 mg	_____	< 300 mg	208 mg

Sources: United States Recommended Dietary Allowances, National Health and Nutrition Examination Survey III

Fewer Calories = Fatter Americans. How can the "ideal" man and woman have higher fat and calorie intakes than the average person? The key is calories—or lack of them. Americans today eat fewer calories than they should to have a healthful food intake. At the same time, there are more overweight people in our country than ever before. In 1980 approximately

25 percent of Americans were overweight, according to government statistics. In 1999 approximately 55 percent of Americans—or 97 million adults—were too heavy.

Fewer calories and fatter people? If you haven't figured it out, the missing puzzle piece is exercise, or rather the lack of exercise. For many, extra pounds pile up because of small, but consistent, imbalances. Just fifty extra calories a day adds up to five pounds a year. In ten years your weight would slowly swell to fifty extra pounds. Of course, these calculations don't take into account that calorie needs decrease with age.

If you're part of the minority who maintain an outwardly normal weight, don't feel smug yet. A normal weight may look good on the outside but doesn't provide a clue to your internal health. The self-assessments in this chapter will.

Deprivation—that's what many people think is required to be healthy. Instead of focusing on what you need to eliminate from your lifestyle, try a new approach. Look at what you're missing and figure out how to add in those things. You have two options for getting started. If you're a person who's highly motivated and ready to take action now—go get a sharp pencil or two—it's time to do some planning. As you read through this chapter, take time to fill in the quizzes and questionnaires right in the chapter to help keep you on track.

On the other hand, if you tend to get bogged down or sidetracked, I encourage you to skim the fill-in-the-blank parts and finish reading the entire book before you begin.

For the Record

Dig out whatever medical records you have on hand. Find out the following before you start:

- blood pressure (systolic/diastolic)
- total cholesterol
- high-density lipoprotein (HDL) and low-density lipoprotein (LDL) cholesterol
- electrocardiogram results, if you've ever had this test

Also, ask your doctor if you've ever had atrial fibrillation (irregular heartbeat in the upper chambers of your heart).

Rate Your Plate

Keep track of everything you eat and drink for the next three days. Research shows this is the best way to determine how you eat. Write it all down. If you need a form to get started, use the one on page 10. A blank checkbook register works better because you can carry it around in your pocket or purse. This task may take some time, but the valuable information you gain will be worth it. It's human nature not to 'fess up to every single thing you eat or drink—but do it anyway. Remember, this record is for you. So don't try to fool yourself. Eat the way you usually do. That will give you the best snapshot of your own style of normal eating. You'll be able to compare and contrast your eating style with today's nutrition recommendations.

NUTRITION **A**CTION Make copies of the form on page 10 or transfer the headings into a check register. Don't depend on your memory at the end of the day. As soon as you finish eating anything, write it down. If possible include at least one weekend day—especially if your eating changes dramatically on weekends.

Sample Food Record Form

Here's a partial example of the level of detail you'll need to include:

How Much	Food or Drink	Time	With Whom/ Where	Accompanying Activity
¾ cup ½ cup	100% bran cereal 1% milk	7:11 A.M.	Kevin, Matthew, Ryan, and Daniel	helping Matthew practice spelling words
½ large	banana	7:23		
6 small	jelly beans	7:40	alone in the car	driving to work
½ cup	water	9:00	Paula at the water fountain	talking
2 slices	extra-thick whole-grain bread	11:50	Julie and Mikki at company cafeteria	talking, looking at photos
2 thin slices (about 1 ounce)	extra-lean ham			
2 tsp.	Dijon mustard			
small piece	iceberg lettuce			
1½ cups	tossed salad made with romaine lettuce, mushrooms, shredded carrot	12:25 P.M.		
3 Tbs.	light ranch dressing			
12 oz.	bottled water—plain	2:00	alone at my desk	making my to-do list

continue like this for the whole day

Write down everything—get picky! Keep track of all beverages, including water, coffee, and diet soft drinks. You're counting more than calories here. Be sure to list seasonings, condiments, and extras. Don't forget the three french fries you snatched from your kid's Happy Meal or the piece of candy from your coworker's desk. They all add up, so write them down. Be as precise as you can about serving sizes. Look on food packages for clues,

YOUR PERSONAL FOOD RECORD FORM

How Much	Food or Drink	Time	With Whom/ Where	Accompanying Activity

such as the total weight of a product. Be especially careful estimating fats such as oils, margarine, and salad dressings. If you eat at quick service or other restaurants, ask if they have nutrition information available on their products. The key is to get as much detail as possible about all that you eat and drink. The quality of your personal food analysis is only as good as the quality of your record keeping.

Next, use your completed food journal as a guide to help answer the following questions. Your answers focus on important areas that don't show up on a nutrient analysis summary. What you write here will give you a quick way to tune in to your eating style and habits.

Personal Nutritional Survey

Who purchases the food in your home? _____

Who prepares it? _____

How many meals do you eat each day? _____

How many snacks? _____

Do you ever skip meals? Which ones? _____

Do you eat alone? How often? _____

What else are you doing besides eating? (working, watching TV, driving, etc.) _____

Do you avoid any foods for health or personal choice reasons? Which ones? _____

How many times each week do you eat foods prepared away from home?

What restaurants do you go to most often? _____

List any medications (over-the-counter or prescribed) you regularly take:

_____

List each supplement, how much you regularly take, and what benefit you are seeking: _____

_____

Do you eat when you're not hungry? When or why? _____

Do you eat too much of any type of food? Which ones? _____

Are there foods you don't eat enough of? Which ones? _____

How often do you consume soft drinks and alcoholic beverages? Which ones? _____

Access the free web site on page 12 so you can enter your food journal into a computerized program that provides detailed feedback on specific nutrients. If you don't have access to a computer, use any of the popular food composition books (*Bowes & Church's Food Values of Portions*

Commonly Used, J. B. Lippincott Co., or *The Most Complete Food Counter,* Pocket Books) and look everything up. This method takes a lot longer, but you'll get similar results. If you go to library for a nutrient composition book, ask if they have any computers online; it will be much faster and more fun. You'll need to know your current height and weight and will be asked to estimate your activity level. Simply key in the basic kind of food on your list and up will pop a detailed selection from which to choose your specific item and amount.

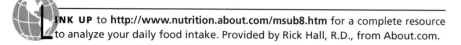

LINK UP to http://www.nutrition.about.com/msub8.htm for a complete resource to analyze your daily food intake. Provided by Rick Hall, R.D., from About.com.

You'll learn what you're doing right and where there's room to make small improvements for big gains in your overall health. In just a few days you can have a clearer understanding of your eating style. This do-it-yourself nutrition analysis won't be nearly as precise as a professionally supervised analysis. So don't hesitate to consult a professional, especially if you are pregnant, have health problems, are at risk for chronic disease, or are following a restricted diet. (See Chapter 10 for information on how to choose a qualified nutrition professional.)

IT'S A FAMILY AFFAIR

Now that we've covered the basic information about your current eating habits, it's time to explore the other factors that impact your health and nutritional status. While you have little control over most of the following concerns, it's important to know your family history as you plan your nutrition strategy.

Nutrition is a balance between environmental and genetic factors. Almost every chronic disease that has a nutrition component also has a genetic component. Studies of families, especially those with twins who are separated at birth, provide strong evidence that genetics affects the development of chronic disease. Sometimes, as with obesity, a family history greatly increases your risk of the same disease. On the other hand, many cancers are the result of environmental conditions, not your genetic makeup.

To help determine your chances of developing a chronic disease, talk with your family. Find out who developed health problems, at what age, and with what outcome. Note clusters of related ailments—heart disease, types of cancer, and so on. Then talk to your doctor. Ask for guidance in evaluating the information you have collected. One case of cancer in your extended family may be just bad luck. But if you find several, then your own personal risk increases. This is especially true if the relatives were in your immediate family or were affected at a young age. If that's your situation, a genetic counselor or specialist might be the most appropriate person to review your history. They might suggest additional tests to more clearly judge your personal risk. For example, there is a new homocysteine test for heart disease, or perhaps you need a baseline mammogram earlier than age 40.

LINK UP to http://www.lifelinks.mb.ca or http://www.randomhouse.com/amahealth/tree for other sample forms and information on how to complete your family medical history.

Shore Up Your Immune System

In the 1990s at least ten top-selling books on nutrition had "immunity" in their titles. You may know that immunity is important to your health, but just what does it have to do with the food you eat? In addition to immunizations to build immunity, it's now becoming clearer that what you eat can make a big difference in how your body fights off disease and protects itself.

NUTRITION ACTIONS

- Take inventory of your medical history, lifestyle, and current eating habits.
- Analyze your food records and complete your personal nutrition survey.

It's hard not to use military adjectives when talking about your immune system. It's mission is to protect and defend your entire body. There are two main branches of your immune system. In the first group are the defenders who provide general service. Defenders fight off everything they encounter to protect you from harm. Your skin, hair, sweat, body oils, saliva, and tears are part of the defense. These immune protectors get physical and set up invasion barriers to protect your internal organs and tissues.

The selective service immune protectors are more highly trained. They launch antibodies that destroy just one type of invader. Then they go on the attack. Together, these specialists are equipped to combat more than 100 billion types of enemies, and they have very long memories. If you've ever been attacked by a particular germ before, they remember and launch an immediate attack.

Having a decreased level of even a single nutrient can weaken your natural resistance to disease. Sometimes your immune system can get shell-shocked. Your defenders spin out of control and start attacking your own body tissues. Lupus is a form of arthritis that is caused by an immune system gone bad. A variety of factors help strengthen and protect immunity. Eating a healthful diet that contains a variety of specific nutrients that can enhance your immune system is essential. A strong immune system can help you stave off many of the health problems we've looked at— in spite of your family history.

DETERMINE YOUR NUTRITIONAL HEALTH

The warning signs of poor nutritional health are often overlooked. Use this checklist to find out if you are at nutritional risk. Read the statements and circle the numbers in the yes column that apply.

For each yes answer you score the number in the box. Total your score to determine your nutritional health.

	YES
I have an illness or condition that made me change the kind and/or amount of food I eat.	2
I eat fewer than two meals per day.	3
I eat few fruits or vegetables or milk products.	2
I drink three or more servings of beer, liquor, or wine almost every day.	2
I have tooth or mouth problems that make it hard for me to eat.	2
I don't always have enough money to buy the food I need.	4
I eat alone most of the time.	1
I take three or more different prescribed or over-the-counter drugs a day.	1
Without wanting to, I have lost or gained ten pounds in the last six months.	2
I'm not always physically able to shop, cook, and/or feed myself.	2

TOTAL = _____

0–2   Good! Recheck your nutritional score in six months.

3–5   You are at moderate nutritional risk. See what can be done to improve your eating habits and lifestyle. Recheck your nutritional score in three months.

6 or more   You are at high nutritional risk. Take this checklist the next time you see your doctor, dietitian, or health care provider. Talk with them about any problems you may have.

Remember that warning signs suggest risk but do not diagnose any medical condition.

Source: Nutrition Screening Initiative

Dietary Evolution

Computers are helping humans gain insights that may help solve today's diet-related health problems. University of Arkansas anthropologist Peter Ungar has found a way to use computer-mapping techniques to chart the landscape of teeth and learn how the human diet might have evolved. Precise computer-calculated numbers chart the grooves in tooth surfaces and indicate how food and liquid might accumulate or drain over the teeth. Human dental fossils mapped with GRASS (Geographical Resources Analysis Support System) help to show what humans evolved to eat. "We didn't evolve to eat cheeseburgers and milkshakes, that's for sure," says Ungar. Human ancestors consumed fewer grains and more fruits and vegetables, getting more protein, vitamins, minerals, and fiber than people in today's affluent societies eat. As humans grew grains, developed alcohol, cultivated sugar, and mined salt, dietary changes began to evolve so fast that our anatomy could not adapt. This relatively rapid change in eating habits has increased many chronic diseases such as cancer, diabetes, high blood pressure, and heart disease.

LINK UP to http://www.cast.uark.edu/local/icaes/conferences/wburg/wburg. html for research summaries from a variety of institutions on diet and human evolution from the International Congress of Anthropological and Ethnological Sciences.

Impact of Food versus Family Genetics

What you eat—and what you avoid eating—can change the odds for or against your long-term health. Optimal nutrition can also help ward off conditions including heart disease, cancer, adult-onset diabetes, hypertension, and osteoporosis.

Your nutritional needs are unique—different from anyone else's. Yet all food follows a similar pathway in each of our bodies. Metabolism is responsible for the digestion, absorption, distribution, transformation, storage, and excretion of nutrients. Metabolism causes lots of extreme variations in nutrient needs in people born with flaws in their metabolic system. Faulty genes are to blame for nutrition-related disorders that range from lactose intolerance, inherited high blood cholesterol, to cystic fibrosis. These types of genetic diseases are called inborn errors of metabolism. Essential enzymes that are missing at birth affect individual nutrient needs. Some of these disorders can be treated by avoiding or restricting particular foods. Others require supplementation of nutrients, sometimes in huge amounts, for improvement.

More subtle genetic variations are now being uncovered. A 1998 *Nutrition Reviews* article reports that genetic diversity causes widely different needs for the nutrient folic acid. Researchers estimate that from 8 to 18 percent of people worldwide have a genetic mutation that raises how much homocysteine is in their blood. High levels of this amino acid mean a higher risk for heart disease, stroke, and blood vessel disease. How much folic acid and vitamins B_6 and B_{12} you need to keep homocysteine levels normal can double or triple if you have the mutated version of this gene.

The challenge of nutrition research today is to identify these minor genetic traits that need customized dietary planning. It's time to move beyond the one-size-fits-all approach. Of the many environmental factors that can tip the odds in your favor or tilt them against you, food may be the most important. Fortunately, it is one of the few variables that you can do something about. It's estimated that good nutrition can reduce the incidence of colon cancer by 75 percent, breast cancer by 50 percent, and cancers in general by up to 40 percent. Dr. John Potter, head of a panel on diet and prevention appointed by the World Cancer Research Fund and the American Institute for Cancer Research, says that even those who have a strong predisposition for a certain disease locked into their genes still have their health risks altered by environmental conditions.

GO FIGURE IF YOU'RE A SUPER TASTER

Sensitivity to bitter taste is an inherited trait. Because many plant poisons have a bitter taste, the ability to identify and reject bitter substances was an evolutionary advantage. Research suggests that these "super tasters" tend to reject foods such as broccoli, grapefruit, and soy. Try this test to see if you are a super taster.

Using a hole punch, punch a hole in the middle of a one-inch square of wax paper. Place the hole on the tip of your tongue. Swab some blue food coloring on the exposed part of the tongue. Using a magnifying glass and a flashlight, count the number of pinkish circles (fungiform papillae). Super tasters will have dozens of papillae; nontasters will have only five or six.

The simple fact that your personal genetic code is unique means that not all people will benefit equally from improving their eating habits. This explains why some people who "do everything right" develop fatal diseases in their 30s and 40s. Remember the extremely untimely deaths of athletes Florence Griffith Joyner and Jim Fixx? On the other hand, almost everyone knows of someone who makes poor food choices, never exercises, smokes, and lives a century or more—like cigar-puffing comedian George Burns.

You can't change who your birth parents are, and for the moment you're stuck with whatever random combination of genes you received from them. Here's a quick summary of the more common conditions that may have a genetic link and how to evaluate your likelihood of developing them. For more specifics on how to improve your odds of preventing or managing one of these chronic conditions, see Chapter 9.

Food Allergies

Eight foods cause 90 percent of all allergic reactions. They are peanuts, tree nuts, shellfish, fish, eggs, soy, wheat, and milk. Allergic symptoms such as hives, tingling lips, and breathing difficulties begin within minutes to one hour after contact with the food. You don't have to eat something to develop an allergic reaction. Schoolchildren allergic to milk can have a reaction if milk is accidentally splashed on their skin. Flying in an airplane can cause someone with a peanut allergy to react. Peanuts don't even have to be served on the flight—the peanut dust in dirty air filters is enough to trigger a reaction.

A severe food allergy is a serious, life-threatening condition. If you find that hard to believe, it's probably because so many people think they are allergic to particular foods. A recent survey showed that up to 25 percent of adults believe they have a food allergy. Scientific studies and testing, however, find that only 1 to 2 percent of adults have a true food allergy. Up to 5 percent of all children have food allergies. Fortunately, most children outgrow their allergies, but nut allergies are usually lifelong.

Although anyone can develop a food allergy, often it's an inherited trait. Children with one allergic parent have about twice the risk of food allergy than children without allergic parents. If both parents are allergic, a child is four times more likely to develop a food allergy than if neither parent is allergic. Most studies show that what a mother eats when she is pregnant has little, if any, effect on sensitizing her child to food allergy. For that reason, it's not recommended to avoid foods during pregnancy that you can otherwise eat and enjoy without symptoms. One exception may be peanut products. It's suggested that women who have allergies or have a close family member with allergies avoid peanuts and peanut-containing products during pregnancy.

On the other hand, breast milk is more likely to sensitize your baby if allergies run in your family. For most infants, breast-feeding has a protective effect against food allergy. Babies fed infant formula are more likely to develop food allergies as infants. It's believed that allergy-susceptible infants who are breast-fed may be sensitized to the tiny amounts of food allergens in their mothers' breast milk. If you or your spouse is allergic, it might be reasonable to avoid highly allergic foods such as nuts and shellfish for as long as you breast-feed your infant.

If you suspect you may be allergic to one or more foods, see a board-certified allergist. Allergists are the only professionals qualified to diagnose and treat most allergies.

You've already collected most of the medical history you need to schedule an appointment. Here are the steps commonly used to diagnose a food allergy:

1. Review the symptoms you experience and figure out your family history for allergies.

2. Evaluate your food records to note if any particular foods seem to trigger reactions.

3. Have a physical examination to rule out other health problems that may be causing your symptoms.

4. Get a skin test: small amounts of suspect food components are injected into your skin to evaluate skin and blood antibody reactions.

5. Go on an elimination and challenge diet supervised by your allergist. First you eliminate the suspect food for several days. Then at the doctor's office you eat that food and are observed for reactions.

INK UP to **http://www.foodallergy.org** for more information on food allergies. The Food Allergy Network also provides a wealth of resources to help people cope with food allergies.

It's important to verify allergies to food so that you don't mistakenly eliminate wholesome foods from your diet without cause. For more information on the difference between food allergy and food intolerance, see Chapter 9.

Cancer—According to the American Cancer Society (ACS), 188,000 of the 564,800 (33 percent) cancer deaths were related to nutrition in 1999. Compare that number to the 175,000 tobacco-related deaths and the 19,000 deaths related to excess alcohol that same year. Several cancers, including many forms of breast and colon cancer, are primarily genetic in origin. But more often cancer develops from the interaction between your genetic code and your environment—which includes what you eat. Although you may inherit a gene for a certain type of cancer, it usually takes some kind of environmental event (smoking, high-fat diet, chemical exposure) to stimulate the growth of precancerous cells. Your genes may load the gun, but it's your food choices and environment that pull the trigger.

Not all cancers have similar roots. Most research suggests that a low-fat diet aids in the prevention of cancer. But women on severe fat-restricted diets (15 percent of calories or less) actually produce more dense breast tissue over time, and dense tissue more frequently develops into cancerous lumps. Don't get frustrated over these contradictory positions. Remember there are few absolutes.

1999 New Cancer Deaths by State

NH	5,400
ME	7,000
WA	23,800
MT	4,100
ND	3,100
MN	19,400
VT	2,600
MA	30,700
OR	15,900
ID	4,600
WY	2,000
SD	3,400
WI	23,700
MI	44,200
NY	83,100
RI	5,200
CT	15,100
NE	7,400
IA	14,300
IN	27,900
OH	56,500
PA	66,600
NJ	40,000
NV	8,100
UT	5,200
CO	13,300
IL	56,800
WV	10,600
DE	3,800
MD	22,600
VA	29,000
DC	3,000
CA	112,300
KS	12,000
MO	27,900
KY	20,500
NC	35,500
AZ	20,000
NM	6,500
OK	15,800
AR	13,800
TN	26,800
SC	17,900
MS	13,000
AL	21,100
GA	29,100
TX	77,400
LA	20,300
FL	88,000
AK	1,400
HI	4,300
PR	

Source: U.S. Department of Health and Human Services, Centers for Disease Control and the Centers for Disease Control Report, "Chronic Diseases and Their Risk Factors: The Nation's Leading Causes of Death," 1999

Diabetes—Both types of diabetes, Type 1 (starts in childhood; always requires insulin) and Type 2 (adult-onset; sometimes requires insulin), have genetic links proven by research of families and twins. There are 625,000 new diabetics diagnosed each year. That's a 10 percent increase in the last decade. More than 80 percent of diabetics die with some form of heart or cardiovascular disease. Adult-onset isn't such an accurate description now that more teens and young adults are developing Type 2 diabetes. More than 80 percent of all diabetes is the adult-onset variety, which is strongly linked to obesity. When you eat too much your pancreas has to overproduce insulin to keep up with your extra food and body mass. At some point your pancreas just wears out or shuts down and can't make enough insulin any more.

As more older women give birth, especially if they are overweight, the rate of developing diabetes during pregnancy (gestational diabetes) rises dramatically. Women who give birth to babies weighing ten pounds or more have a much higher risk for developing diabetes themselves. Babies born to mothers who had diabetes during pregnancy are more likely to have health problems later in life themselves.

Classic research with the Pima Indian tribes in Mexico and Arizona shows the dramatic influence that lifestyle can have on health. Both Mexican and Arizona Pimas are descendants from the original Pima tribe. The Mexican Pimas still eat traditional staples such as corn, beans, and fruit. Very few Mexican Pimas are overweight and diabetes is rare. Pimas who live in Arizona eat a typical American diet that is high in both sugar and fat. Many Pimas from Arizona are overweight. As a result, it's normal for these Pimas to develop diabetes by the time they are 55.

Heart Disease—Fewer Americans are dying each year from heart disease, but the number of people with first heart attacks has held steady or even increased since 1987. In a study reported in the September 1998 *New England Journal of Medicine,* Wayne Rosamond from the University of North Carolina says the decrease in deaths is most likely due to better treatment for people once they have a heart attack, not from prevention.

Don't skip this section if you're female. Coronary heart disease is the single largest killer of American women. More women than men die from heart disease every year. Two times as many women die from heart disease than from all types of cancers combined. If you're a woman between the ages of 45 and 64, it's critical to have your blood cholesterol tested. That's the age range where most women's cholesterol increases from under 200 to an average of 217 to 235.

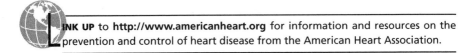

LINK UP to http://www.americanheart.org for information and resources on the prevention and control of heart disease from the American Heart Association.

Heart disease claims at least half a million lives every year and contributes to soaring health care costs. It restricts the activities of thousands who develop the disease in midlife. You can delay or prevent the onset of heart disease by changing the way you eat. Choosing more fruits and vegetables can lower both cholesterol and blood pressure. Food modifications alone cannot overcome the ill effects of smoking, high blood pressure, being overweight, and not exercising, but they can help you live better and longer.

The following checklists will help determine your probable risk for heart diseases compared to others your age. They're a combination of scientifically tested ratings. If you're under 30 or over 74 , there isn't enough research to predict your age-related risk.

RATE YOUR RISK FOR HEART DISEASE

1. Record the point score for your age and sex.   _____

Men	Age	Women
−1	30–34	−9
0	35–39	−4
1	40–44	0
2	45–49	3
3	50–54	6
4	55–59	7
5	60–64	8
6	65–69	8
7	70–74	8

2. Find the point score for your LDL cholesterol level.   _____

Men	LDL	Women
−3	below 100	−2
0	100–159	0
1	160–189	2
2	190 or higher	2

3. Find the point score for your HDL cholesterol level.   _____

Men	HDL	Women
2	below 35	5
1	35–44	2
0	45–49	1
0	50–59	0
−1	60 or higher	−2

4. Find the point score for your blood pressure.   _____

If your systolic and diastolic pressures are in different categories, use the point score from the higher category. For example: 115/82 = 0 points for both men and women.

Men	Systolic/Diastolic	Women
0	below 120/below 80	−3
0	120–129/80–84	0
1	130–139/85–89	0
2	140–159/90–99	2
3	160 or higher/100 or higher	3

5. Find your point score for other risk factors.   _____

Men	Risk Factor	Women
2	Do you have diabetes?	4
2	Do you smoke?	2

Total up your points. _____

Note: Be sure to subtract negative points.

Your risk of getting heart disease in the next ten years is:

Men	Total Score	Women
1%	less than −2	1%
2%	−2	1%
2%	−1	2%
3%	0	2%
4%	1	2%
4%	2	3%
6%	3	3%
7%	4	4%
9%	5	5%
11%	6	6%
14%	7	7%
18%	8	8%
22%	9	9%
27%	10	11%
33%	11	13%
40%	12	15%
47%	13	17%
56%	14	20%
	15	24%
	16	27%
	17 or more	32%

Compare Your Risk

Okay, so how do you compare with the average person your age? Use the following chart to see if your risk rate is better or worse than others your same age.

Note: "Low-risk" people don't smoke or have diabetes. Their blood pressure is 130/85 or lower. Their LDL is 100 to 129 and their HDL is 45 or more for men and 55 or more for women.

Average-Risk Men	Low-Risk Men	Age	Low-Risk Women	Average-Risk Women
3%	2%	30–34	less than 1%	less than 1%
5%	3%	35–39	less than 1%	less than 1%
7%	4%	40–44	2%	2%
11%	5%	45–49	4%	3%
14%	8%	50–54	6%	5%
16%	12%	55–59	7%	7%
21%	12%	60–64	9%	8%
25%	13%	65–69	11%	8%
30%	14%	70–74	14%	8%

Source: Adapted from Framingham Heart Study Data in *Circulation,* 1998

Note: The people in the Framingham study were mostly white, middle-class men who lived in a Boston suburb. If you aren't white or middle class, your risks could be higher or lower. Since not many women over 55 were included in this study, the risks for older women are probably much higher than these numbers indicate. Other risk factors that are too hard to measure, such as family history, levels of exercise, and obesity, were not included, but probably show up in other areas, such as blood pressure or having diabetes. Remember, there are no perfect studies or evaluation methods.

High Blood Pressure—Almost half of all people with high blood pressure have a parent with high blood pressure, too. About 10 percent of our population has blood pressure that increases when they eat too much sodium. Since more African Americans than Caucasians have this sensitivity, it may be linked to genes.

Environmental factors, including smoking and diet, are estimated to influence half your risk of developing this silent killer. Eating ten servings of fruits and vegetables is as effective as prescription drugs in lowering high blood pressure. Before you roll your eyes and wonder how you could possibly eat ten servings every day, take a look at the following mix-and-match chart.

Mix and Match Your Ten a Day

Fruit or Vegetable	Servings
12 oz. glass fruit juice	2
8 oz. glass vegetable juice	2
½ cup canned or frozen fruit	1
1 large piece fresh fruit	2
lettuce and tomato (on a sandwich)	1
½ cup cooked or raw vegetables	1
large dinner salad (2 cups lettuce)	2
vegetable-topped pizza (1 slice)	1
fruit juice Popsicle	1
fresh fruit (to top frozen yogurt)	1

Obesity—The majority of the adult U.S. population—97 million adults—is overweight or obese. The rate of obesity has risen from 25 percent of adults in 1980 to 55 percent in 1999. These alarming statistics are even worse for low-income populations, especially for poorer women.

It's not just Americans who are getting fatter. According to the World Health Organization Consultation of Obesity, in 1998 the global projections on obesity for the next decade are so serious that action is urgently required. Obesity is today's most neglected public health problem.

FAT OF THE LAND

Other countries where more than 25 percent of the adult population is obese include: Brazil, Chile, Colombia, Costa Rica, Cuba, Kuwait, Mexico, Morocco, Peru, Samoa, and Tunisia.

Willpower and self-control have little to do with the ability to maintain a healthy weight. At least six factors influence your weight—behavior, environment, health status, culture, income level, and genetics. Most people who are overweight had at least one overweight parent. If both your parents were overweight, it's highly likely you will be overweight or constantly struggling to maintain a healthy weight. Metabolism may be partly determined by your genetic makeup. Some people are also genetically prone to store extra fat on certain parts of their bodies. If you're not overweight but have thick thighs or chubby cheeks, blame your ancestors.

Research hasn't shed much light as to why some people tend to gain weight so easily, while others never stray from their ideal weight. Medical researchers are making strides in identifying the causes of obesity. On the other hand, most common solutions for weight management fail miserably.

The Excessive Fat and Consumption Trends in Obesity Risk (X-FACTOR) survey says only 30 percent of obese adults report that a doctor has encouraged them to diet for health reasons. Even a minor loss of 5 to 10 percent body weight can dramatically improve health for those who are overweight. If you weigh 200 pounds (and if 150 is your ideal weight), losing just 10 to 20 pounds could lower your high blood pressure, send your cholesterol level back to normal, or allow you to stop medication to control your blood sugar levels.

Go **FIGURE**—How Do You Shape Up?

Your body mass index (BMI) is a way to judge your body weight in relation to your height. The National Institutes of Health (NIH) says BMI is the best initial rule of thumb for judging if you weigh too much. If you are amazingly fit and well muscled or under 5 feet tall or younger than 18 or over 70, this test won't work for you. For the rest, it's just what the NIH said—an initial way to consider the health of your shape.

Calculate Your Body Mass Index (BMI)

$$BMI = \frac{(W \times 705) \div H}{H}$$

W = your weight in pounds

H = your height in inches

19 or less:	Underweight, may suggest malnutrition or serious disease
25–20:	Healthy weight
25–27:	Overweight
27–30:	Overweight, with moderate health risk especially if you have a weight-related health problem or a family history of high blood pressure, heart disease, and/or diabetes
over 30:	Obese, with severe health risk for weight-related problems above, plus osteoarthritis, stroke, and some forms of cancer

Do You Have a Hazardous Waist?

LINK UP to http://www.bodymassindex.com or http://www.mealformation.com/bmassidx.htm for an automatic BMI calculation and lots of helpful information on judging the state of your shape.

Need an easier way to check if your body is up to par? Just wrap a tape measure around your middle near your belly button. A waist measurement of 35 inches or more in women and 41 inches or more in men means you probably have too much tummy fat. Abdominal fat is a more serious threat to your health than fat stored elsewhere. Almost all your vital organs are housed between your shoulders and waist, and extra fat here changes hormone levels, alters insulin production, and makes your organs work extra hard. Fat pads on your hips, thighs, or rear end don't have the same dramatic health effects.

Selected Studies

Women overweight in the abdominal area are at increased risk for coronary heart disease. An eight-year study followed 44,702 women, aged 40 to 60. Women with a waist-to-hip measurement ratio of .88 or more were 3.25 times more likely to have coronary heart disease than women with a ratio of .72 (*Journal of the American Medical Association*, vol. 280, 1998). Waist-to-hip ratio is determined by dividing your waist measurement by your hip measurement (e.g., 32 ÷ 4 = .8). This research shows that regardless of BMI, the risk for heart disease skyrockets for women with too much tummy fat.

Body fat isn't all bad. It's like a soft polar fleece wrap that keeps your body temperature constant and protects vital organs. Without enough fat, brain development in children decreases and sex hormones don't work well. Teenage girls who are too lean often have delayed puberty. Too little body fat for too long can lead to permanent infertility in young women. Overzealous parents who impose fat restrictions on children under the age of 2 can irreversibly stunt the growth of their children's bodies and minds.

 LINK UP to http://www.shapeup.org to access former surgeon general C. Everett Koop's web site on weight control. Be sure to visit the cyberkitchen and the fitness center.

LINK UP to http://www.caloriecontrol.org for overall diet and fitness information from the Calorie Control Council.

Osteoporosis

The woman in the doctor's waiting room is 35 years old, but her bones are like a 47-year-old woman's. She looks and feels like a healthy young woman, but she's suffering from osteoporosis. What you eat as a teenager has a direct impact on the strength and density of your bones as you age. Other factors play a role, but foods rich in calcium are key to the prevention of osteoporosis.

Short women with northern European ancestors have a higher rate of osteoporosis than any other group. Osteoporosis is a disease that gradually weakens your bones and often leads to painful fractures, including hip fractures. For many people with osteoporosis, a broken hip results in a fall, not the other way around.

Early diagnosis of bone loss is important because you lose more bone as you age. Osteoporosis is a silent risk factor. You don't feel anything as a result of your weakened bones—until you break your hip, back, or wrist. Bone fractures resulting from osteoporosis are not only disabling, they can be life-threatening. According to C. Conrad Johnston, Jr., M.D., vice president of the National Osteoporosis Foundation, "Twenty percent of people die in the year following a hip fracture."

LINK UP to http://www.nof.org to get the cutting-edge reports on new research and treatments for osteoporosis from the National Osteoporosis Foundation.

Osteoporosis Risk

What are your chances of developing brittle bones? Check off your risk factors below. Five or more high-risk answers increase the likelihood of osteoporosis.

Risk Factors	High Risk	Low Risk
Sex	Women	Men
Race	White or Asian	All others
Age	Over 45	Under 45
Weight	Thin, underweight, or frail	Normal or overweight
Exercise	No regular exercise or only swimming	Regularly exercise, especially weight-bearing activities like walking, bicycling, aerobics, and tennis
Smoking	Yes	No
Alcohol consumption	Drink 2 or more alcoholic beverages per day	Don't drink alcohol or drink 1 or fewer per day
Eating foods rich in calcium (1,200 mg day = 4 cups milk)	No	Yes
Family history of osteoporosis	Yes	No

The more checks you have in the high-risk categories, the greater your overall risk for developing osteoporosis. You can improve more than half of the risk categories with permanent lifestyle changes.

If the results from this checklist show you have a high risk for osteoporosis, ask your doctor to order a bone density test. This is the only sure way to determine the strength of your skeleton and estimate your risk for fracture. The tests (there are several methods) are all painless and easy. Your bone density, after it has been measured or calculated, is compared to age-matched normal samples of bone.

Selected Studies

Researchers studying the ongoing bone mineral density and risk of fractures in 207 mother-daughter pairs have shown a strong genetic link for osteoporosis. There is a strong correlation between the height, weight, and body composition of these mother-daughter pairs that may contribute to the inheritance of bone density (*Journal of Bone and Mineral Research,* January 1999). Osteoporosis prevention and early intervention is critical for women with a positive family history of this disease.

 ANDY HOTLINE To find a bone density testing center near you, a service of the National Osteoporosis Foundation Action Line, call 1-800-464-6700.

Stroke

Strokes strike lightning fast without warning—just a split-second feeling that something has gone very wrong. The problems that cause stroke, however, are years in the making. Eating lots of fruits and vegetables, controlling your weight, and drinking skim or low-fat milk may reduce your risk from this killer.

A stroke is like a heart attack in your brain. Blood vessels in your brain can develop plaque and clots just like those in your heart and other parts of your body. When a major blood vessel to the brain is blocked, the part of your brain nourished by that blood vessel dies. Though it's not included in the following risk assessment, women who use oral contraceptives are much more likely to have a stroke than those who don't use birth control pills.

Recent study findings have suggested that risks for stroke or heart attack rise in the hours following a high-fat meal. That's because an overload of fat affects the ability of arteries to dilate in response to changes in blood flow during digestion. For that reason it's important to pay attention to how you eat over time but also to what you eat in a single day or a single meal.

RATE YOUR RISK FOR STROKE

You need to be 54 or older to score this quiz.

1. Record the point score for your age.   _____

Age	Points
54–56	0
57–59	1
60–62	2
63–65	3
66–68	4
69–71	5
72–74	6
75–77	7
78–80	8
81–83	9
84–86	10

2. Record your point score for your systolic blood pressure.   _____

    Note: If you take medicine for high blood pressure, this
    should be your systolic blood pressure while on medication.

Systolic BP for Men	Points	Systolic BP for Women
95–105	0	95–104
106–116	1	105–114
117–126	2	115–124
127–137	3	125–134
138–148	4	135–144
149–159	5	145–154
160–170	6	155–164
171–181	7	165–174
182–191	8	175–184
192–202	9	185–194
203–213	10	195–204

3. Find your total point score for other risk factors.   _____

Men's Points for Yes	Risk Factors	Women's Points for Yes
2	Do you have diabetes?	3
3	Do you smoke?	3
6	Have you ever had an electrocardiogram that shows you have an enlarged heart muscle (left ventricular hypertrophy)?	4
3	Have you had one or more of any of the following?	2

- heart attack

- chest pain during physical activity

- severe leg pain on exertion that results from an inadequate blood supply (intermittent claudication)

- the symptoms of a heart attack, but no increase in the enzymes that show muscle damage

- congestive heart failure symptoms including breathlessness and severely swollen ankles caused by your heart's failure to pump enough blood and oxygen

4. Find your point score if you take medication to lower your blood pressure. _____

   Note: If you do not take medication, your score is 0.

   Men who take medications for high blood pressure score 2 points.

   Women use the chart below:

Women's Systolic Blood Pressure on Medication	Points
95–104	0
105–124	1
125–134	2
135–154	3
155–164	4
165–184	5
185–204	6

Rate Your Risk

Men	Points	Women
3%	1	1%
3%	2	1%
4%	3	2%
4%	4	2%
5%	5	2%
5%	6	3%
6%	7	4%
7%	8	4%
8%	9	5%
10%	10	6%
11%	11	8%
13%	12	9%
15%	13	11%
17%	14	13%
20%	15	16%
22%	16	19%
26%	17	23%
29%	18	27%
33%	19	32%
37%	20	37%
42%	21	43%
47%	22	50%
52%	23	57%
57%	24	64%
63%	25	71%
68%	26	78%
74%	27	84%
79%	28	
84%	29	
88%	30	

Compare Your Risk for Stroke

Compare your risk of having a stroke to that of an average person your age.

Men	Age	Women
3%	55–59	6%
5%	60–64	8%
7%	65–69	11%
11%	70–74	14%
16%	75–79	18%
24%	80–84	22%

Source: Adapted from Framingham Heart Study Data
published in *Circulation*, 1998

Note: The people in the Framingham study on stroke were mostly white, middle-class men who lived in a Boston suburb. If you aren't white or middle class, your risks could be higher or lower. Since not many women over 55 were included in this study, the risks for older women are probably much higher than these numbers indicate. Other risk factors that are too hard to measure, such as family history, levels of exercise, and obesity, were not included, but probably show up in other areas, such as blood pressure or having diabetes. Remember, there is no perfect study.

LINK UP to http://www.strokeassociation.org for stroke information and http://www.americanheart.org for an interactive assessment guide and stroke information from the American Heart Association.

The next few chapters showcase why eating healthful foods is such a smart thing to do. You'll find out how it's the balance of nutrients in foods that make some eating styles better than others. Once you understand the complexities of the nutrients in the foods you eat, it's easier to appreciate why balance, variety, and moderation are keys to improving your odds for a long and enjoyable life.

2

You Are What You Eat: A Nutrition Primer

N ew nutrition is a process, not specific actions. New nutrition is an attitude about food that is positive and enthusiastic. New nutrition is more than getting the minimum you need to avoid deficiency. It's the enjoyment of choosing, preparing, and eating wholesome foods that taste good and are satisfying. Your food choices should concentrate on foods that are your best health investment. New nutrition includes foods that provide emotional comfort, too, so don't eliminate your favorites. Learn to appreciate them in moderation if they have too much or too little of what you need.

Eat foods as close to their natural state as possible. A fresh apple is more nutritious than applesauce. Applesauce is a better choice than apple pie. Savor the flavor and sensations of the foods you eat. Slow down and make eating an event instead of a chore. Enjoy the process of learning about the new nutrition—it tastes great! Remember, it's your total eating habits over time that matter most. Decisions on individual foods should be made with this in mind.

ARE YOU IN THE KNOW ABOUT H₂O?

Why start a chapter on food with a discussion of water? Water is the basis of life. Your body is nearly two-thirds water, making it the most important nutrient. You can survive for long periods of time without calories, protein, carbohydrate, fat, vitamins, and minerals. Without water, you won't last more than a few days.

It's estimated that two-thirds of Americans fall at least 1 quart shy of getting their daily ½ gallon requirement of water. You typically lose 2 to 3 quarts of water each day through breathing, sweat, urine, and feces.

Do you make the common mistake of waiting until you're thirsty before taking a drink of water? Thirst isn't an early signal of water needs; it's a warning sign that you're dehydrated and need to drink—and fast. By the time you feel thirsty you have already lost about 1 percent of your

Body of Water

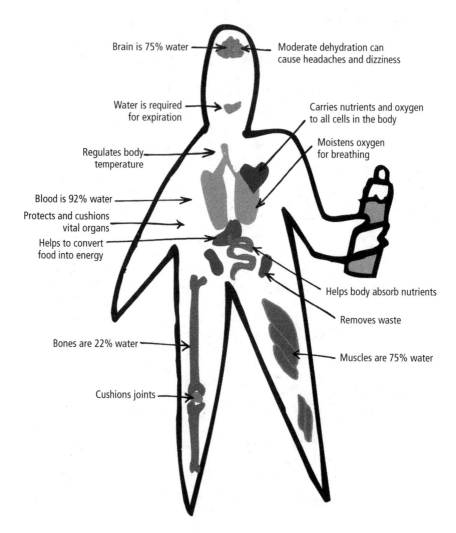

Brain is 75% water — Moderate dehydration can cause headaches and dizziness

Water is required for expiration

Carries nutrients and oxygen to all cells in the body

Moistens oxygen for breathing

Regulates body temperature

Blood is 92% water

Protects and cushions vital organs

Helps to convert food into energy

Helps body absorb nutrients

Removes waste

Bones are 22% water

Muscles are 75% water

Cushions joints

total body water. Some subtle signs of dehydration include dry lips, dark-colored urine, muscle or joint soreness, headaches, crankiness, fatigue, and constipation. More serious complications caused by extreme dehydration include seizures, permanent brain damage, or even death.

In addition to water, milk, juice, and soup count toward your daily fluid intake because of their high water content. But don't include alcohol, coffee, nonherbal tea, and soft drinks that contain caffeine, as they may have a mild diuretic effect. Caffeine can hold back water from the tissues that need it. Since your body is nearly two-thirds water, it is important to stay ahead of dehydration. If you are out in hot, humid weather or are exercising vigorously, you need to replace 150 percent of the amount of water lost to keep hydrated. If you lose 1 pound of sweat during a workout (16 ounces), you need 24 ounces of fluid to rehydrate. The message is crystal clear: Drink plenty of water every day.

Go **Figure**
It's been estimated that you can use only 54 percent of the water from a diet cola. Bladder cancer risk drops 7 percent for every 8 ounces of water you drink.

Nutrition Actions to Increase Water Intake
- Take water breaks instead of coffee breaks.
- Choose water instead of soft drinks or coffee.
- Drink water before meals and snacks.
- Drink water before, during, and after any physical activity.
- Keep a bottle of water on your desk to sip from throughout the workday.
- Alternate sparkling or plain bottled water with alcoholic drinks at parties and social gatherings.

The critical role of water in maintaining personal health has made the safety of public drinking water a national issue. Disease from untreated water is virtually nonexistent in the United States, but natural disasters such as floods, earthquakes, or accidental contamination of wells or municipal water supplies can be devastating. Beginning in 1999, all local water utilities were required to send citizens a report on the safety of the local tap water. At a minimum your report should tell you where your water comes from, levels of pollutants, and if these levels violate Environmental Protection Agency (EPA) regulations. Most important, the report should include a plan to correct any problems. Some water quality reports are incomplete or indecipherable. If you don't understand your report, get help.

Handy Hotline Call the EPA's water hotline at 1-800-426-4791.

Link up to http://www.epa.gov/safewater for more information on how to find out the rating of your local water supply from the Environmental Protection Agency.

Is Bottled Better?

Water is classified as "bottled water" or "drinking water" if it meets all applicable federal and state standards, is sealed in a sanitary container, and is sold for human consumption. Bottled water cannot contain sweeteners or chemical additives (other than flavors, extracts, or essences) and must be calorie-free and sugar-free. Flavors, extracts, and essences—derived from spices or fruit—can be added to bottled water, but these additions must comprise less than 1 percent (by weight) of the final product. Beverages containing more than the 1-percent flavor limit are classified as soft drinks, not bottled water. In addition, bottled water may be sodium-free or contain very low amounts of sodium. Some bottled waters contain natural or added carbonation.

Recently, the safety of bottled water has been called into question. The National Resources Defense Council (NRDC) released a study in March 1999 that concluded some bottled water is not necessarily cleaner or safer than most tap water. However, only a small fraction of the 103 brands tested had problems. Many of the brands that failed the NRDC tests were grocery-store gallon jugs and very small local bottlers. However, most U.S. bottlers voluntarily belong to the International Bottled Water Association (IBWA) that requires more stringent testing and regulatory levels than federal or state rules. In addition, members of the IBWA, who produce about 85 percent of the bottled water sold in the United States, must meet strict industry standards established by the association. These standards, contained in the IBWA "Model Code," exceed the FDA regulations currently in place for bottled water. According to the Centers for Disease Control and Prevention (CDC), bottled water has never been responsible for an outbreak of waterborne illness.

LINK UP to http://www.bottledwater.org/public/ibwp_facts_reg.htm if you want all the details on bottled water regulations from the International Bottled Water Association.

NUTRITION ACTION Since disasters usually happen without warning, keep a few days' supply of bottled water stored for emergencies. Estimate ½ gallon per person each day for drinking water and an additional ½ gallon for cooking, washing, and first aid.

CALORIES: A CONTROL ISSUE

Your body uses the energy from the foods you eat to support basic bodily functions and physical activity. This energy comes in the form of calories. Your calorie needs change many times over the course of a lifetime. Infants and teens need the most calories per pound to help meet increased demands during growth spurts. Pregnant women also have increased need for calories, especially during the later months of pregnancy and if they breast-feed their baby. People who are active, do manual labor for a living, or exercise frequently need more calories than people who aren't physically active. Calorie needs also shrink some with age. Regardless of how many calories you need, your need for important nutrients doesn't shrink. That's why it's harder for inactive people to get enough nutrients from food.

Go Figure

3,500 calories = 454 grams = 1 pound

1 gram = $\frac{1}{28}$ ounce = the weight of 1 small paper clip

1 gram protein = 4 calories = $\frac{1}{3}$ small egg white

1 gram carbohydrate = 4 calories = $1\frac{1}{2}$ teaspoons apple juice

1 gram fat = 9 calories = scant $\frac{1}{4}$ teaspoon olive oil

1 gram alcohol = 7 calories = 1 ounce beer, 1 tablespoon wine, or $\frac{1}{2}$ teaspoon 100-proof distilled spirits

One ounce of beer has more than the 7 calories that alcohol provides—it also contains calories from carbohydrates. The energy or calorie content of a food depends on the combination of nutrients it has. In theory, it takes 3,500 extra or unused calories to equal 1 pound. If you eat an extra 500 calories a day for a week, you should gain 1 pound if your activities remain constant. Too many calories above what you need for energy will make you fat.

Just look around—more than 55 percent of all Americans are overweight. At any given time one-fourth of men and almost half of all women are trying to lose weight. The solution isn't lower-calorie diets. We already eat fewer calories in the United States than almost ever before in our country's more than two-hundred-year history. The typical American woman doesn't eat enough calories to get the minimum levels of nutrients needed for health. Researchers at the USDA discovered it's next to impossible to eat enough nutritious foods on limited-calorie diets. In *Ideas for Better Eating: Menus and Recipes to Make Use of the Dietary Guideline from the USDA* (1981), top nutritionists tried to create meal plans that would meet the USDA Dietary Guidelines and RDAs at varying calorie levels. The bottom level was to be 1,200 calories. It couldn't be done—even by the experts. It takes a minimum of 1,600 calories worth of nutritious food to meet the recommended minimum levels of vitamins and minerals. A 1,600-calorie intake doesn't allow for many extras like alcohol, soft drinks, and candy.

The solution? Activity. We just don't move enough. Modern conveniences have pushed physical activity out of our lives. How many phone extensions and remote control devices do you have in your home? Have you ever driven by a health club and watched people circle the parking lot for ten or more minutes trying to find a close spot? Heaven forbid we have to walk more than a few steps to enter the building for an aerobics class. If you want to have a healthful eating style, you need to burn enough calories to be able to eat a reasonable amount of food.

LINK **UP** to http://www.cdc.gov for the first ever surgeon general's report on physical activity and health that includes recommendations for regular moderate physical activity from the Centers for Disease Control.

HANDY **HOTLINE** for the Centers for Disease Control's nutrition and physical activity information line is 1-888-232-4674 (CDC-4NRG).

Calories and Common Sense Still Count

Calories are more than a system to determine how fattening a particular food is. A calorie is a unit of energy that you either use or store. You add calories by eating food. You subtract calories by what you do—breathing, walking, talking, even digesting food! The balance between what you eat and what you do determines how much you weigh and your level of health.

Too often we think of balancing the calorie equation by cutting back on food intake. It's time to refocus on the other side of the equation—the output or expenditure of calories. Back in the 1950s, renowned nutritionist Dr. Jean Mayer suggested that Americans were gaining weight not because we were eating too much, but because we weren't moving enough. Other experts thought he was way off base. Today, there is mounting evidence that Dr. Mayer was right. Small differences in how much we work our bodies may be a primary cause of obesity.

The Burning Truth

Not all activities burn calories at the same rate. Exercising harder or faster for a given activity will only slightly increase the calories you expend. A better way to use up more calories is to exercise longer at the same intensity. Lighter people burn fewer calories doing the same activities as heavier people.

If you keep your food intake constant and decrease your daily physical activity by 500 calories, you should gain a pound in one week (7 days × 500 calories = 3,500 calories = 1 pound). But research from the University of Vermont shows that it's not quite that simple. Excess calories from fat are more fattening than extra carbohydrate calories. Your body has a limited capacity to change carbohydrate into body fat, but the sky is almost the limit when it comes to storing fat calories. If you eat 100 excess calories from fat, 97 of them will be converted to body fat. If your 100 surplus calories came from carbohydrate, only 77 would turn to fat. The rest would be used for energy.

Average Calories Burned in 20 Minutes of Continuous Activity

	125 pounds	150 pounds	175 pounds
Light housework (washing dishes, folding clothes, cooking)	35	45	50
Raking leaves, gardening	60	75	85
Heavy housework (scrubbing floors, vacuuming, carpentry)	65	80	95
Cycling (6 mph)	65	80	95
Walking (3 mph)	85	110	125
Mowing the lawn (push mower)	110	135	160
Aerobic exercise (dance, kick boxing)	125	150	180
Swimming (continuous laps)	140	165	190
Cross-country skiing	195	235	270
Climbing stairs	235	280	335
Jogging (7 mph)	255	310	360

On the activity side of the equation, there are discrepancies, too. The less lean muscle tissue you have, the fewer calories you need to maintain your weight. If two people weigh exactly the same, but have different proportions of muscle and fat, they will need different amounts of calories to perform the same activities. A well-muscled person needs more calories per pound than someone who has a high proportion of body fat. When you diet (cut calories) to lose weight, at least 25 to 30 percent of the weight you shed isn't fat but water, muscle, bone, and other lean tissue. That's true regardless of what type of food plan you choose. The less muscle in your body, the lower your metabolic rate—and the harder it will be to lose fat and keep it off.

There is no single, easy way to accurately calculate your calorie needs. How much energy you spend in a given task or activity can vary considerably. The amount of energy you expend doing the same work (mowing the lawn, shoveling snow) changes day to day.

GO FIGURE your calorie needs. A quick estimate of your energy needs is:

1,600 calories—many women and older adults

2,200 calories—children, teenage girls, active women, most men

2,800 calories—teenage boys, active men

Note: pregnant or breast-feeding women usually require more calories that those listed for women or active women.

LINK UP to http://www.healthstatus.com/calorieburn.htm to calculate your individual calorie requirements at the HealthStatus assessment site.

CARBOHYDRATES: KEEP THEM COMPLEX

There are two types of carbohydrates: simple and complex. Both types are found almost exclusively in plant foods. Simple carbohydrates are sometimes called simple sugars. The more important complex carbohydrates are also called starches.

Complex carbohydrates are the premium grade of fuel for your body's energy needs. That's because carbohydrates are easily stored in your muscles. These complex carbohydrates break down more slowly than simple sugars and release their available glucose over time. Most nutritionists agree you should eat more complex carbohydrates and less fat and simple carbohydrates.

Did you ever try this experiment in high school science class? Put a small piece of unsalted soda cracker on your tongue. Keep in it your mouth, without chewing, for several minutes. All of a sudden you will begin to notice a sweet taste. That's because carbohydrate digestion has already started in your mouth. Salivary enzymes change the long chains of complex carbohydrates into shorter glucose (or sugar) chains. While they digest rapidly, complex carbohydrates take longer to break down than simple carbohydrates and give you a greater feeling of fullness when you eat.

Simple carbohydrates are (as the name suggests) much less complex, and that makes them easier to be digested and utilized as a quick source of energy. Foods that are high in simple sugars usually have few, if any, naturally occurring vitamins or minerals. Examples of simple carbohydrates include white sugar, brown sugar, honey, soft drinks, hard candy, and various sugars that are added to many processed foods. Fruit juice, because it does not contain the fiber found in fresh fruit, also acts like a simple carbohydrate. Simple sugars become a problem when you eat too many of them instead of more nutritious foods.

Diets rich in complex carbohydrates can increase your brain level of the amino acid tryptophan, which is converted to serotonin, a calm-down, feel-good chemical. Some people, especially women, may tend to crave carbohydrate foods for the antidepressant effect that high levels of serotonin provide.

PROTEIN: YOUR HANDYMAN

Protein is your body's do-it-yourself handyman. Protein helps to build and maintain just about everything in your body. From muscles to membranes and blood vessels to bones, protein helps make it and keep it in good repair. Different proteins have different jobs. Keratin helps form hair, nails, and the outer layer of your skin. Actin, myosin, and myoglobin form the meaty part of muscle. The "globin" (GLOW-bin) part of hemoglobin is the protein that fills the rubbery inside of your bones, including the marrow.

Proteins are made up of structural units called amino acids, of which there are twenty-two. Nine of these amino acids you can only get from foods. They are called the essential amino acids (leucine, lysine, isoleucine, tryptophan, threonine, methionine, valine, phenylalanine, and histidine). Your body makes the other thirteen amino acids when needed. All twenty-two amino acids link together to form chains. It's like playing Scrabble; you work with the letters you have to build onto base words. Similarly, you need to eat foods containing just the right essential amino acid to fill each link in the body's amino acid chain to make it complete.

Amino acids can be found in many foods, but animal foods have the highest and most complete assortment. Beans, lentils, and grain products also have some protein, but vegetable foods have less total amino acids and fewer combinations of the essential ones. Vegetarians may remember the days when they were advised to eat "complementary proteins." We now know that you don't have to combine foods at mealtime to make complete proteins. Eating an assortment of nonmeat protein foods over the course of a day does just fine.

Most Americans eat more protein than they need. Although it's important to get enough protein, too much can be hard on your kidneys and make them work overtime. Too little protein isn't desirable either. Skimping on protein can leave you sluggish and prone to infection. Protein is an energizing nutrient. If you've been seriously ill, injured, or have had major surgery, your body needs extra protein, calories, and other nutrients for repair and recovery. If your handyman doesn't have the right tools, he can't do the job.

FOCUS ON FAT

A St. Paul firefighter, on the verge of retirement, was required to attend my nutrition class as part of on-the-job continuing education. The topic was how to lower blood cholesterol levels. He was clearly not interested (this was in the 1970s). He alternated muttering snide comments and snoring during the presentation. At the end of class he blurted out, "Miss, I don't believe anything you just said. My old uncle Joe had a farm, and every day for breakfast he ate a half dozen fried eggs, bacon, and sausage and poured real cream in his coffee. For lunch and supper his wife served fried meat and poured gravy over the whole plate. They ate pies and used butter on everything. His diet was loaded with fat and he lived to be 99 and died peacefully in his sleep." It was a dietitian's dream-come-true to respond to him. "What you said makes perfect sense," I began. "I'll bet your uncle Joe led a heart-healthy lifestyle. He lived at a time when farmers did hard labor for ten or more hours a day. [Remember this nephew was at retirement age in the 1970s.] They didn't have the benefit of air-conditioned tractors and labor-saving devices in the early 1900s. It wasn't unusual for farmers to burn 10,000 or more calories a day. College football players in training easily eat that much today. If you need 10,000 calories to meet energy needs, you can eat as much as 333 grams of fat a day and still be on a low-fat diet. Just think of all the other nutritious foods you could consume with the remaining 6,000+ calories!"

For years the message has been to eat less fat. Now the reality is beginning to look considerably more complicated. The controversy over fat has leapt out of the frying pan and into the fire. For more than a decade we have been fixated on types of fat and fat grams. Some people are drastically cutting back on fat and at the same time eating more calories and gaining weight. Fat was named the culprit for practically every chronic disease. Now scientists are taking a closer look. Maybe fat isn't so bad. After all, it's an essential nutrient needed for good health from cradle to grave.

Fats are really combinations of many different fatty acids, and each one differently affects how your body works. With nine calories per gram, fat is the most concentrated energy source in food. Fat is critical for growth in children, is required for healthy skin, helps hormonelike substances regulate body processes, and is essential for the absorption of fat-soluble vitamins.

Average fat intake in America is down from 36 percent of total calories in the period 1976 to 1980, to 34 percent based on data from the 1988 to 1991 National Health and Nutrition Examination Survey (the most recent data available). Don't celebrate yet! The percentage of total calories from fat has declined, but actual fat intake has increased from 81 to 83 grams per day. The reported drop in percentage of calories from fat is the result of slightly higher calorie intakes, not improved diets. Eating more calories without increasing physical activity is not the ideal way to decrease the percentage of calories from fat, unless exercise is increased.

Have you ever felt that just thinking about fatty foods makes you fat? Your instincts may not be off base. A study at Purdue University tested the effects of tasting high-fat foods on blood fat levels. Two varieties of cream cheese were the variables. One cream cheese was full fat and the other fat free. The people in the test were asked to hold some cream cheese in their mouth and not swallow. They actually had to spit it out. The level of triglycerides in the blood was measured both before and right after their taste. Those who had the full-fat cream cheese had significantly elevated triglyceride levels compared to those who had the fake, fat-free stuff.

Top Ten Fat Sources in Adult American Diets

Men	Women
Mixed dishes and combination foods in which meat, poultry, or fish are primary ingredients	Mixed dishes and combination foods in which meat, poultry, or fish are primary ingredients
Mixed dishes and combination foods in which grains are primary ingredients	Mixed dishes and combination foods in which grains are primary ingredients
Beef, not in mixtures	Table fats like butter or margarine
Hot dogs, sausages, and luncheon meats	Beef, not in mixtures
Table fats like butter or margarine	Milk, other than nonfat
Milk, other than nonfat	Hot dogs, sausages, and luncheon meats
Salad dressings	Salad dressings
Fried potatoes and potato chips	Cookies, cakes, and pies
Cookies, cakes, and pies	Cheese, not in mixtures
Cheese, not in mixtures	Bread

Source: Continuing Survey of Food Intakes by Individuals, 1989–1991

Types of Fat

The first time people really started thinking about the fat in their diets wasn't until the 1960s and 1970s. In fact, cholesterol was the first villain, not fat. Then saturated fat was deemed the bad guy. For the first time many consumers started reading the ingredient lists for products they routinely bought. They learned that "animal" fats were bad and "vegetable" fats were good. Until that time, many of the newer convenience products like cake and baking mixes contained lard.

When consumers found lard and other animal fats in their favorite products, they were upset. As a result of major consumer backlash, most food companies quickly dropped saturated fats and replaced them with hydrogenated vegetables oils. Fast-food restaurants also made the switch from cooking french fries in beef tallow to frying in hydrogenated vegetable oils. While "hydrogenated vegetable oils" may sound better than lard, they are *worse* for your overall health. That's because hydrogenated fats not only raise levels of harmful cholesterol (LDL), these fats reduce the amount of the protective, good cholesterol (HDL).

Fats are combinations of different fatty acids. Foods that contain fat may have combinations of three or four different fatty acids. You may have heard that olive oil is a monounsaturated fat. It really is a combination of monounsaturated, polyunsaturated, and saturated fatty acids. Olive oil's most predominant fatty acid, however, is monounsaturated.

Rate Your Fat Habits

Circle the answer that best corresponds to your usual eating habits, then tally your score to see how your fat intake rates.

Do you:	Rarely	Sometimes	Often
Drink 1% or skim milk?	0	5	10
Add butter or margarine to bread, potatoes, or vegetables?	10	5	0
Use nonstick pans or cooking sprays instead or oils or solid fats?	0	5	10
Usually snack on regular chips, cookies, crackers, cheese, or nuts?	10	5	0
Use more than 1 tablespoon of regular (or 2 tablespoons of low-fat) salad dressing at a time?	10	5	0
Eat regular hot dogs, luncheon meat, or sausage more than once a week?	10	5	0
Remove extra fat from meat and skin from chicken before eating? OR If you don't eat meat, do you use reduced-fat cheeses and nut butters?	0	5	10
Balance high-fat foods with low-fat choices during the day?	0	5	10
Choose meals that include french fries when you eat out?	10	5	0
Eat pastries and doughnuts for breakfast or snacks?	10	5	0

Scoring

- 0–45   It's time for some changes. Look for reduced-fat versions of your high-fat favorites.
- 50–80   You're on your way but need a little fine-tuning. Review your food records and make notes of where you can cut the fat.
- 85–100   Keep up the good work. Don't get obsessive about fat—remember, it is good for you in moderation.

Fat Effects: The Good, the Bad, and the Ugly

X = undesirable effect	Trans	Saturated	Poly- unsaturated	Mono- unsaturated
HDL Cholesterol (GOOD)	lowers X	raises	lowers X	neutral
LDL Cholesterol (BAD)	raises X	raises X	lowers	neutral
Total Cholesterol (UGLY)	raises X	raises X	lowers	neutral

Monounsaturated—Because monounsaturated fats aren't damaged by oxidation, they are less likely to increase cholesterol buildup in your arteries. *Mono* is the Latin word for "one." That means monounsaturated fatty acids have one double bond. The more bonds a fatty acid has, the more saturated or stable it is. Monounsaturated fats tend to break down more readily than saturated fats. They are best used for salad dressing, stir-frying, and sautéing. Because most monounsaturated fats come from nuts, seeds, or olives, they add distinct flavors to foods. Some of the most common sources of monounsaturated fat include olives and olive oil, canola oil, peanuts and peanut oil, walnuts, sesame seed oil, and avocados.

Selected Studies

A Swedish study of more than 61,000 women between the ages of 40 and 76 collected data on eating habits and other risks for breast cancer. Researchers found that replacing other types of fat with monounsaturated fat cut these women's risk of breast cancer by 45 percent (*Archives of Internal Medicine*, January 1998). While most studies focus on olive oil, this study suggests that the protective benefit lies with monounsaturated fats as a whole category of food, rather than specifically with olive oil.

Polyunsaturated—This fat is liquid at room temperature; its structure has two or more double bonds, thus giving the name "polyunsaturated" (*poly* means "many"). Research suggests that these fats lower blood cholesterol if they are substituted for other fats in a low-fat diet. Most polyunsaturated oils are odorless and can withstand high temperatures. They work well for deep-fat and pan frying, general baking, and cooking. Best sources include corn, cottonseed, soybean, safflower, and sunflower oils.

Saturated—This fat is usually solid at room temperature and has no double bonds in its structure. Research suggests that particular saturated fatty acids can increase blood cholesterol. Saturated fats also raise the good (HDL) cholesterol, and that is a positive benefit. Look for the grams of saturated fat on the nutrition facts label of the food you buy. The main sources of saturated fat include animal fats and coconut and palm tree oils.

Trans—Trans fats are processed by taking an unsaturated fat (like oil) and adding hydrogen to its chemical makeup to make it saturated, stable, and solid at room temperature. Research suggests that these fats increase blood cholesterol and should therefore be limited. You'll find trans fats in almost all restaurant fried foods and most commercial cookies, cakes, frostings, crackers, snack foods, and chips. Margarine, while it suffered the brunt of the criticism about trans fatty acids, it not a major source compared to the other foods mentioned.

Trans Fatty Acid Content of Foods

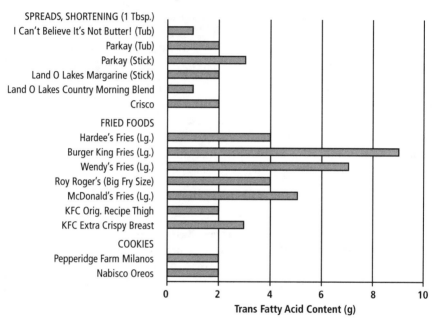

Trans Fatty Acid Content (g)

FIBER

Fiber is the part of a plant that cannot be digested by human enzymes. Fiber is found in vegetables, fruits, whole grains, and legumes. Because fiber is not digested, it provides no calories or energy. It does provide bulk that helps move waste quickly through your intestinal tract.

Whole grains, such as wheat, oats, barley, rye, and brown rice, retain all the parts of the grain kernel after milling. There are three components to grains: endosperm, bran, and germ. The endosperm stores most of the carbohydrate and protein and some B vitamins and fiber. The tough bran coating houses more than two-thirds of the B vitamins, minerals, and fiber found in grains. The germ (the embryo that develops to form the new plant) contains polyunsaturated fat and vitamin E. Refined grains keep only the endosperm. Enriched grains add back just some of the vitamins and minerals lost during processing.

Go Figure your fiber needs

Most experts recommend you aim for 1 gram of fiber for every 100 calories you eat. That translates to 25 grams of fiber for 2,500 calories, and 30 grams for 3,000 calories. Even if you eat less than 2,500 calories, 25 grams a day is considered the minimum.

Use a different formula to calculate fiber needs for children. "Age + 5" is the rule to follow. A 2-year-old should have no more than 7 grams of fiber and a 10-year-old up to 15 grams daily. Children should not have fiber-added products or fiber supplements. Too much fiber in the diets of growing children can decrease appetite and increase nutrient losses.

There are two main types of fiber: soluble and insoluble. They have different but important functions. Some foods contain both types of fiber.

Soluble Fiber—dissolves in water and forms a gummy substance similar to liquid rubber cement. These gums bind cholesterol and carbohydrates in your intestines, and that decreases blood sugar and circulating cholesterol. The best sources of soluble fiber include barley, dried beans and peas, fruits (especially apples, apricots, figs, mangoes, oranges, peaches, plums, rhubarb, and strawberries), lentils, oat products, psyllium, vegetables (especially broccoli, brussels sprouts, cabbage, carrots, okra, sweet and white potatoes, and turnips).

Insoluble Fiber—nature's whisk broom, sweeps out unwanted debris. It doesn't dissolve in water, but it acts like an intestinal sponge soaking up water and expanding the bulk of waste products (feces). That makes stools softer and easier to move through your intestines. Insoluble fiber speeds up the time waste is in your digestive tract and helps to prevent constipation, hemorrhoids, and diverticulosis. Soft but bulky stools that move quickly also decrease your chance of developing rectal and colon cancer. Hard stools can injure the delicate walls of your large intestine. Since waste material contains what your body doesn't want or need, a speedy exit is desirable. The longer waste stays in you, the more direct contact you have with harmful bacteria and toxins. The best sources of insoluble fiber include bran cereals, brown rice, corn and popcorn, fruits (especially apples, berries, pears), vegetables (especially asparagus, beets, carrots, kale, okra, peas, sweet and white potatoes, spinach), 100 percent whole-grain breads, and pastas.

Since both types of fiber require water for processing, it's essential to stay well hydrated. If you increase your fiber intake, you need to drink more water, too. Increasing physical activity is also recommended as you increase fiber because it helps stimulate muscle tone necessary for speedy elimination.

Nutrition Actions to Get Your Fiber Fix

Befriend Beans—rich in fiber and protein, try packaged instant beans, reduced-fat refried canned beans, or other canned beans. Build meals around bean dishes and add to salads and soups.

Go for Grains—look for 100 percent whole-wheat or whole-grain bread and check fiber grams on food labels.

Feast on Fruit—eat a piece of fruit instead of drinking juice or eat dried fruit as a snack.

Put Away Your Peeler—Eat the skins of potatoes and other fruits and vegetables, just be sure to wash them well first.

Boost Breakfast—Mix a high-fiber cereal (more than 5 grams of fiber a serving) with your regular brand and top with fruit.

Skip the Chips—Eat crackers with 2 grams of fiber per ounce instead of chips and serve with a chickpea dip such as hummus instead of creamy dips.

Most people aren't willing to count calories, add up fiber grams, or figure percentages every day. It takes too much time and effort. Yes, the basics in this chapter are important, but strapping a calculator to your wrist isn't the way to make food decisions. Change your view of food. Instead of seeing how many calories or fat grams are in a particular food, look for the benefits. Choose foods based on their positive attributes, such as colorful produce that's bursting with flavor and nutrients or hearty whole-grain breads. Eat like a gourmet and savor every bite. There's more to food than its nutritional value; it's an essential part of the social side of life. Try to make meals an event instead of a mad dash. It does take more planning time to have optimal nutrition, but it's worth it physically and emotionally. Don't get bogged down in the numbers; they're only a reference point—use them that way.

3

Foods in the News

What does food have to do with health and happiness? More than we ever imagined. Hidden within foods are hundreds of compounds that take the food-health connection to an exciting new level. Mother Nature planned a clever way to protect her luscious bounty. Smelly sulfur compounds in onion and garlic act as a natural insect repellent. Other plant chemicals, or phytochemicals, protect vegetation from harmful bacteria and viruses. When you eat foods that contain these plant-protecting compounds, they begin to protect you, too. Instead of providing insect resistance, they work to halt the forces that zap health in humans such as cancer, high cholesterol levels, and can even slow the aging process. Foods from animals can also play a role in maintaining and promoting health. Their special mix of nutrients provides some of the richest combinations of protein and minerals.

Foods are not perfect. Eat too much of anything and it will probably make you sick. That's why the habitual nutrition advice of balance, variety, and moderation has never gone out of style. When it was first discovered that ingredients in foods can cause cancer, the reaction was to identify and remove all carcinogens from food. But that's not possible—too much of anything could probably cause cancer. Today's advice is to eat a greater variety of foods and to be active enough so you can consume plenty of foods and thereby have access to the huge variety of compounds that can promote health and longevity.

THE GOOD NEWS: FROM AVOCADOS TO ZUCCHINI

There is no one miracle food that has everything you need. For that we should be thankful, because variety is the spice of life. In fact, if you rely on the same boring repertoire of foods, you probably don't have a nutritious diet. Some food surveys show that many Americans eat a grand total of about twenty different foods. That's not only boring, it's bound to be unhealthy. Variety is a key component of new nutrition. Here's a sampling of some recent, newsworthy food items (remember that good nutrition never goes out of style, even if certain foods do).

Amazing Avocados

With more than five hundred varieties to choose from, it's stunning to think that Americans are familiar with only two types of this fruit. Haas avocados from California are small in size and very dark green with a thick bumpy skin. For the same amount of avocado, the Haas variety has more than double the fat and calories of the second variety, the Florida avocado. The Florida version is much bigger and has a brighter, smoother green skin. Most of the fat in both types is monounsaturated. However, the Haas avocado contains up to one-third of its fat from saturated fat. You'll also find fiber, vitamin A, niacin, folic acid, magnesium, and potassium in all avocados.

Beans, Beans, They're Good for Your Heart

We've gotten the message to eat more dried beans and peas. In 1974 the average American ate just 5.5 pounds of legumes each year. In 1994 we were up to 7.3 pounds per person per year. There's still room for improvement. Beans are a heart-healthy food—they do help lower cholesterol and reduce the rate of heart disease. The soluble fiber in beans acts like a sponge, soaking up cholesterol and mopping it out of the way. Beans can also help stabilize blood sugar levels and reduce your risk of breast or prostate cancer.

Yes, there are unpleasant side effects associated with bean consumption—flatulence or gas. On average, most people pass gas about fifteen to twenty times every day. A variety of foods besides dried beans can cause gas, such as bran, broccoli, and cabbage.

NUTRITION ACTIONS TO FEND OFF FLATUENCE

Try these tips to help reduce potentially embarrassing emissions.

- Soak beans before cooking and be sure to use fresh water for cooking.
- Build your bean intake slowly. Give the bacteria in your digestive tract time to adjust to processing those complex carbohydrates.
- Consider a gas-reducing aid (like Beano) that helps break down the complex carbohydrates in beans before they can ferment in your colon.

What's the Beef over Beef?

Beef has gotten a bad reputation in recent years for being high in fat and cholesterol, and ground meats may carry food-borne illnesses like *E. coli*. Lean portions of meat can help prevent nutrient deficiencies, boost your immune system, and build stronger blood. Moderation is the key. Researchers for the American Council on Science and Health (ACSH) investigated claims that vegetarian diets are better for you because they eliminate meat. According to Dr. Ruth Kava, ACSH director of nutrition, "The mere fact that a diet is meatless does not guarantee that it is healthful. And although eliminating meat is a way to reduce saturated fat and increase plant foods in the diet, it is not the only way. Balance, moderation, and variety are the keys to a healthy eating plan." The researchers found that vegetarians tend to make more healthful lifestyle choices, such as regular exercise; they maintain a desirable weight; and they don't smoke, abuse alcohol, or use illegal drugs. Current thinking is that it's not the absence of meat but the presence of lots of whole grains, fruits, and vegetables that make an eating style healthful.

Selected Studies

A three-site clinical trial comparing the effects of lean red meat and lean white meat on blood cholesterol levels is the third study to conclude that lean red meat, as part of a healthful diet, can help lower blood cholesterol levels. The study included 191 men and women who followed a basic low-fat diet. The half who used lean red meat had similar reductions in low-density lipoprotein cholesterol (LDL—the bad stuff) and elevations in high-density lipoprotein cholesterol levels (HDL—the good stuff) (*Archives of Internal Medicine*, June 1999). If you enjoy red meat, there's no reason to ban it from your diet; just choose lean cuts like round and loin.

Biotech Benefits

Do you eat cheese? If so, you're a consumer of the benefits of biotechnology. Over half of the rennet used in cheese-making is produced through a biotech fermentation process that eliminates the "old-fashioned" method. (If you've read Laura Ingalls Wilder's *Little House on the Prairie* books, you'll remember that to make cheese, a baby calf had to be sacrificed for the rennet found in its stomach lining.) Rapid-rise yeast products that speed up bread-making were developed in England by rearranging and duplicating certain yeast genes. Imagine french fries that absorb less fat, crops designed to resist bugs without insecticides, and plants rich in nitrogen without the use of chemical fertilizers. This isn't science fiction. Each of these ideas is being worked on right now. Some, like insect-resistant crops, are already a reality.

Early humans were hunters and gatherers who ate only what they found or could successfully hunt. Eventually they figured out how to grow certain plants as crops. For ten thousand years people have been using genetic science to improve crops and create new food products. Selecting seeds, baking bread, brewing beer, fermenting fruit into wine, and making cheese are all examples of harnessing biology to make and modify plants and food products. Some of these methods have become quite sophisticated over time.

Traditional plant crossbreeding helps improve on the random cross-pollination naturally provided by birds, bees, and other insects. It typically takes ten to twelve years to sort out and breed a plant that has the characteristics desired in a new variety. The International Food Information Council (IFIC) describes it this way: "When two whole plants are crossed, each having some 100,000 genes or so, all the genes from both plants get jumbled together. Since breeders want only one or a few, this presents a big headache. It's like wanting to add a certain French word to the English dictionary and having to combine the entire French and English dictionaries—just to add that single word."

Modern biotechnology is much more selective. Crop breeders can actually identify and select the precise genetic trait they want and move it into another plant. It's like having a tool that can instantly zero in and find a needle in a haystack. The prime benefits of biotechnology are a more healthful environment and less reliance on harmful chemicals. Some examples:

- Better-tasting, vine-ripened tomatoes year-round. Most tomatoes are picked while green and then chemically ripened with ethylene gas to turn red. Biotechnology eliminates the need for chemical gassing.
- Pesticide and insecticide reduction through plants bred to ward off destructive insects and resist harmful bacteria and viruses. Farmers who use seed that produces resistant plants can cut back or even eliminate their use of chemical herbicides, pesticides, and insecticides. That means less toxic exposure to farm workers, the soil, and water.
- Improved nutrient content of foods to help reduce world hunger and malnutrition. For example, increasing the levels of lysine in rice can reduce the number of children in China who develop blindness as a result of lysine amino acid deficiency. Africans who rely on sweet potato crops for survival lose over half of their crop each year to feathery mottle virus. Biotechnology has bred a sweet potato resistant to this disease that not only dramatically increases production, but also reduces the use of chemicals.
- Biotechnology is expected to positively impact food production by allowing for heartier crops that can withstand drought and flooding or better tolerate extremes of heat and cold. Almost half of the $12 billion American farmers spend on fertilizer each year evaporates or washes away. High nitrogen– absorbing plant varieties may be able to reduce the need for fertilizers and help protect our environment.

Selected Studies

Results from several years of consumer research indicate that most consumers would purchase new fruits and vegetables available through the use of biotechnology. The limiting factor that makes people resistant to biotechnology is lack of education. Less-informed people were more resistant to biotechnology than those who understood the science behind it (*Cereal Foods World*, 1998). If biotechnology concerns you, learn more about it.

Pick Some Blueberries

Blueberries are a perfect example of a fruit with hidden qualities. A quick look at the nutritional analysis doesn't show much to get excited about. But the health benefits of eating blueberries may be as far reaching as preventing cancer and retarding the effects of aging—particularly loss of memory and motor skills. Anthocyanins and other natural compounds are the key. These chemicals are responsible for the intense blue color of the berries.

Selected Studies

According to new research done at the Jean Mayer USDA Human Nutrition Research Center on Aging at Tufts University, blueberries have the highest antioxidant capacity of forty tested fruits and vegetables (*Journal of Agricultural and Food Chemistry*, 1998). Choose deep blue or wild blueberries because they have the highest concentration of ellagic acid, the active ingredient in this fruit.

Canola from Canada

Canola is the combination of two words, Canadian and oil. Canola is a genetic variation of rapeseed developed specifically for its nutritional qualities by Canadian plant breeders through traditional plant breeding techniques. Canola contains the lowest level of saturated fatty acids of any vegetable oil and is high in monounsaturated fatty acids. Like all vegetable oils, canola oil is cholesterol-free.

Capsaicin—It's Hot

The fiery heat you feel from hot peppers is from a pungent compound called capsaicin (cap-SAY-shun). Hot peppers are a natural and instant decongestant and expectorant—they make your eyes and nose run. Capsaicin (also called Substance P), most concentrated in the white membranes of the pepper, is released by your body when you eat hot peppers. It's a chemical that sends pain and itch signals to the brain. There is some evidence that capsaicin may lower cholesterol and help prevent stomach ulcers.

Chocolate: Food or Drug?

Researchers have wondered for a long time what in chocolate generates such a craving. Is it the fat in chocolate, the sugar, the caffeine, or what? Anandamide, a chemical in chocolate, is a naturally occurring substance produced by brain cells that mimics the mental effects of marijuana.

Get Unstuck with Cranberries

Drinking cranberry juice is a common home remedy for urinary tract infections. Not until the late 1990s did anyone figure out why cranberry juice is so effective. It was thought to acidify the urine, but new research says that what really happens is that specific compounds in cranberries inhibit *E. coli* bacterial cells from sticking in the urinary tract.

Selected Studies
Dr. Amy Howell of Rutgers University in New Jersey estimates that the amount of condensed tannins in a 10-ounce glass of cranberry juice taken on a daily basis could help prevent urinary tract infections (*New England Journal of Medicine,* October 1998).

Eggs Are Okay

It's the amount of cholesterol in your blood, not in your omelet, that contributes to risk for heart disease. Mounting scientific research shows that cholesterol from food has just a slight impact on blood cholesterol levels in most healthy people. "There's no connection between cholesterol in food and cholesterol in the blood," says world-renowned nutrition and fat expert Dr. Ancel Keys.

Selected Studies
Harvard researchers have debunked the myth that you should reduce egg consumption if you want to lower blood cholesterol and prevent coronary heart disease. In two large prospective cohort studies of men and women, they found no overall association between egg consumption and risk of heart disease or stroke (*Journal of the American Medical Association,* April 1999). These findings suggest that eating an average of one egg per day (seven eggs per week) won't increase the risk of heart disease or stroke for healthy adults who do not have diabetes.

Fishing for Health

Two or three servings of fish every week is good for your health. The average North American has just one serving of fish weekly. For optimal benefits choose cold-water fish including mackerel, herring, sardines, salmon, and trout. Even though these fish have more fat than others, they're packed with healthful omega-3 fatty acids.

The benefits of eating seafood rich in omega-3 include:

- promoting proper development of brain, nerve, and eye tissue during pregnancy and infancy
- lowering the risk of heartbeat abnormalities that may result in sudden heart attack or death
- prolonging life after a heart attack by improving heart function and reducing damage from heart disease

- modestly lowering blood pressure, thereby reducing the risk of heart attack and stroke
- improving symptoms of certain inflammatory diseases such as arthritis and psoriasis

As with other types of fat, you can't just add to what you already eat. Use fish to substitute for other fatty foods you usually consume, such as processed or fat-riddled meats and fried foods. Usually these foods have more total fat and much more saturated fat than fish. For information on fish oil capsules, see page 156.

Unfortunately, you do need to be concerned about contaminants fish pick up from living in polluted waters. Eating raw fish or shellfish puts you at risk for food-borne diseases, especially parasites, or in the case of mollusks, bacteria or viruses.

NUTRITION ACTIONS: BUYING FISH

- Find a local fish or grocery store that gets regular shipments of high-quality fresh and/or flash-frozen fish.
- Look for signs of freshness, including bright clear eyes, reddish gills, and shiny scales that stick to the fish's skin.
- Take a whiff; there shouldn't be a strong "fishy" odor when raw or cooked. A strong smell indicates decay or bacterial contamination.
- Ask what's freshest and buy it if you're not committed to a certain variety.
- Choose smaller rather than larger fish—they've had less exposure to chemical pollutants.

Flaxseed Each Day Keeps the Doctor Away?

Flax is a blue flowering crop with oil-rich, tiny seeds that range in color from light to reddish brown. The Babylonians cultivated flaxseed as early as 3000 B.C. for linen textiles, and in 650 B.C. Hippocrates used flaxseed for the relief of intestinal discomfort. Today it's common in products such as multigrain cereals and snack foods. Flax adds a pleasant, nutty flavor to foods. With the rise in popularity of bread shops, it is possible to buy fresh bread that contains flaxseed (check the ingredient list). Over half the fat in flax comes from healthful omega-3 and omega-6 fatty acids. Flax is also a good source of both soluble and insoluble fiber. It has seventy-five times more lignin than any other plant food. It is found mostly at co-ops; be sure to ask for milled flaxseed. You can also grind flax at home in a mini–food processor. The seeds must be broken to reap the benefits. Studies show that consumption of flaxseed improves bowel regularity and maintains blood glucose levels. Flaxseed appears to protect against certain types of cancer, particularly hormone-sensitive cancers such as breast, endometrium, and prostate. New research also suggests that alpha-linolenic acid, an omega-3 fatty acid which is abundant in flaxseed, offers protective effects against both coronary heart disease and stroke. Omega-3 has been shown to also protect against hypertension and inflammatory and auto-immune disorders.

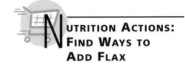

NUTRITION ACTIONS: FIND WAYS TO ADD FLAX

- Add flaxseed to baked goods.
- Sprinkle broken flaxseed over yogurt, cereal, and salads.

Garlic—Crushed Hopes?

Garlic advocates make some potent claims. Hundreds of studies on garlic have been completed in the past ten years alone. The trouble is that many of these studies aren't very good. Some had no control group, others had too few people to draw conclusions.

Garlic, along with onions, leeks, and shallots, are part of the lily family. It's been a staple food and medicine for thousands of years. Egyptian slaves who built the pyramids ate garlic to increase their stamina. Garlic has been used both inside and outside the body to treat everything from viruses to vampires. Garlic was commonly used in both world wars to help ward off infection on the battlefields. The word *garlic* comes from the Anglo-Saxon "gar-leac," or spear plant.

The chemical that gives garlic its strong smell is allicin (from the Celtic language meaning "hot" or "burning"). This unstable compound is released only when the garlic clove is bruised, chewed, or crushed. Allicin then breaks down into other sulfur-containing compounds. Some scientists believe that the allicin is what's beneficial in garlic; others disagree. The Center for Science in the Public Interest (CSPI) tested various garlic supplements and concluded that people should consume fresh garlic or garlic powder instead of garlic pills or capsules. One-third teaspoon of garlic powder contains as much or more allicin than some best-selling supplements. One fresh garlic clove is equivalent to ⅓ teaspoon of garlic powder.

Selected Studies

A study at the University of California at Irvine showed allicin is unlikely to survive in the digestive tract and would be destroyed within minutes of entering your bloodstream (*Journal of Agricultural Food Chemistry,* January 1997). If that's true, it's highly improbable that allicin can accomplish anything at the cellular level. Of course, some compound other than allicin might have the beneficial effects—but no one has found it yet.

The good news is that garlic can't hurt. The American Herbal Products Association's *Botanical Safety Handbook* rates garlic, also considered an herbal medicine, class 2c for safety (not to be used while breast-feeding). The worst it will do is cause digestive upset in sensitive persons. Garlic is perhaps the best example of how little we really know or understand about the chemistry of foods and their relation to health.

Grape Juice—No Wine Here

If you want the reported benefits of drinking wine, without the alcohol, grape juice is the choice for you. Grape juice was originally invented as a nonalcoholic substitute for communion wine during prohibition. It contains the same flavonoids as red wine. The catch is you need to drink more to get the same levels. According to grape juice researcher John Foltz from the University of Wisconsin at Madison, it takes a 12-ounce glass of 100 percent pure grape juice (not grape drink) to provide the same benefits found in 4 to 5 ounces of wine. Keep in mind that 100 percent grape juice is a concentrated source of energy providing 20 calories per ounce, so a 12-ounce glass has 240 calories.

Grapefruit—Red Is Richer

There are lots of myths about this tart, tropical treat. It doesn't burn calories or melt fat away. The grapefruit diet isn't magical. It's low in calories, requires exercise, and replaces the usual variety of fruits with lots of grapefruit. Grapefruit is a great food. It's high in vitamin C and low in calories, and the fiber helps fill you up. If you like grapefruit, choose the red or pink varieties—they contain lots more lycopene than white grapefruit. Lycopene may reduce the risk of certain cancers.

But pill takers beware; don't take your medicine with grapefruit juice! Grapefruit juice can interfere with some medications and increase the dose you absorb. Naringin in grapefruit juice turns off an enzyme in your small intestine that works to metabolize certain drugs. When a drug is not absorbed at the normal rate, more or less of it gets into your bloodstream. This makes the dose different than the amount prescribed and changes the drug's effect. The drugs that most frequently react with naringin include calcium channel blockers that control high blood pressure; Seldane, an allergy medication; and Halcion, an antianxiety drug.

Honey—The Bitter Truth

Honey, like all other sugars, is a sweetener. It provides calories but little in the way of nutrients. Of course, beekeepers and honey producers vehemently deny this fact. One tablespoon of honey provides 60 calories—all from carbohydrates. A tablespoon of sugar has 45 calories. Although honey contains some vitamins and minerals not found in sugar, they aren't significant in the amount of honey usually consumed. You'd have to eat 1½ cups of honey to get even 10 percent of any nutrient other than carbohydrates. That much honey has 1,500 calories and provides more than 140 percent of your total carbohydrate needs for the day.

If you use less honey than sugar to sweeten your coffee or tea (it has a higher sweetening power than white sugar), you've eaten fewer empty calories and that's good. However, honey is sticky sweet and, if not brushed off your teeth, it can promote tooth decay faster than other sugars, including white and brown sugars. Never feed babies less than 1 year old any form of honey, including honey graham crackers or other products made with honey. Honey can contain deadly botulism spores that immature digestive tracts can't handle.

Honey's unique composition of sugar and high acidity makes it useful for treating minor burns and scrapes. Antimicrobial agents in honey, such as propolis found in nectar, can halt the growth of certain bacteria, yeast, and molds. The high sugar content helps pull water out of cuts and sores. Since germs need water to grow and multiply, they don't fare as well when honey is used to dry them up. Sometimes honey can be used to help constipation because its water-drawing action can move needed fluid into your bowels.

Irradiation: If It's Good Enough for Astronauts . . .

Since the 1970s, U.S. and Soviet astronauts have been enjoying irradiated foods in space. It's actually preferred over other food preservation technologies. Food irradiation technology in the United States began as part of the "Atoms for Peace" program established by President Eisenhower. Food irradiation is a food safety tool. Ionized energy (gamma rays, electron beams, or X rays) is applied to foods to eliminate harmful bacteria without the use of heat. Sometimes irradiation is called "cold pasteurization." More than forty types of foods have been approved for irradiation around the world.

Irradiation doesn't make food radioactive. The energy levels used during irradiation are far too low to induce radiation. The process is similar to light passing through a glass window. Food is moved through an energy field and never touches the energy source. Irradiation damages food nutrients far less than basic cooking or microwaving.

Federal regulations require that most irradiated foods be identified with the radura (RAH-dur-ah) symbol accompanied by the words "treated with irradiation" or "treated by irradiation." Currently meat, poultry, fruits, vegetables, grains, spices, seasonings, and dry enzymes used in food production have been approved for irradiation.

Selected Studies
What's the benefit of irradiated meat? Low doses of radiation can kill at least 99.9 percent of salmonella in poultry and an even higher percentage of *E. coli* in ground beef (*Journal of the Institute of Food Technology,* January 1998). This scientific summary encourages the use of irradiation technology to help improve the safety of the food supply.

Nuts to You

It might seem nutty at first, but evidence is building that fat-filled nuts may be beneficial in reducing blood cholesterol levels and protecting against heart disease. While all nuts contain fat, about 85 percent of the fat is polyunsaturated and monounsaturated. It is thought that these unsaturated fats may help to lower "bad" LDL cholesterol.

When you add nuts to your diet, be sure to cut back on fat elsewhere. Research suggests the benefits are obtained only if you replace foods high in saturated fats (such as fried foods and fatty meats) with nuts. You can't just add them in. Nuts are an excellent source of fiber, vitamin E, magnesium, zinc, selenium, copper, potassium, phosphorus, biotin, riboflavin, niacin, and iron. Some nuts are also good sources of folate. In addition to vitamins and minerals, nuts also contain beneficial plant chemicals that help protect you from a variety of chronic diseases.

Olive Oil—What a Fat!

All oils—olive or otherwise—contain the same amount of calories (120) and fat grams (14) per tablespoon. When you replace the saturated fats you eat now with monounsaturated fats, such as those found in olive oil, you might reap health benefits. To gain improvements such as lower blood cholesterol and added protection against heart disease, you can't just add olive oil. You also have to cut back on other fats and oils.

Light or extra-light olive oil does not mean light in calories! Instead light refers to the very subtle flavor of this oil. Light olive oil is an "all-purpose" oil that can be used in everyday cooking without affecting flavor. All olive oils are classified by the amount of acidity, flavor, color, and aroma they impart. The European Economic Communities (EEC) set the standards. Olive oil is more expensive than most vegetable oils. That's because olive oil manufacturing is more labor intensive from harvest to production. Most olive oil producers don't use cheaper, speedier modern processes such as heat extraction and chemical solvents. The higher price of certain olive oils reflects both quality and flavor.

Although olive oil does not require refrigeration, it does lose quality when exposed to heat and light. Many food experts prefer to keep olive oil refrigerated. While chilling may cause some clouding, it doesn't affect the oil's flavor or quality. Any cloudiness will disappear when the oil is returned to room temperature.

Psyllium—It's Husky

Plantain plants from India are the source of psyllium husks. It's the husk portion that is known for its high-soluble fiber content and that is used in food and some over-the-counter laxatives. Soluble fiber, along with a low-fat diet, can lower blood cholesterol. Psyllium husk has fourteen times more soluble fiber than oat bran. The Kellogg Company has recently introduced psyllium-enriched foods including pastas and cereals.

Soft Drinks Edge Out Milk

Twenty years ago, teenagers drank twice as much milk as pop. Now they drink twice as much pop as milk. This intake of soft drinks significantly lowers intake levels for calcium and other key nutrients. Teen girls who regularly consume soft drinks take in 20 percent less calcium than non-drinkers. This lower calcium intake contributes to broken bones now and osteoporosis later. Obesity has risen in tandem with soft-drink consumption, which for many teens accounts for 15 to 20 percent of their daily calories.

NUTRITION ACTION For the lunch hour meal (which now averages twenty-four minutes), add low-fat cheese to sandwiches and salads, eat a cup of low-fat yogurt, or drink a glass of milk. Most convenience and grocery stores sell milk in containers for immediate, single-serving consumption.

Joy of Soy

Soy products are the only food that contains genistein (JEN-iss-tyne). This compound helps stop the growth of tumors and can lower cholesterol in those with high levels in their blood. Soybeans also contain a unique group of phytochemicals called isoflavones which are commonly called phyto-estrogens. Much of the interest in soy estrogens and how they might relieve menopausal symptoms began with a single report published in the January 1998 *Obstetrics and Gynecology Journal.*

According to the 1997 National Report on Consumer Attitudes about Nutrition, 50 percent of Americans thought that soy was healthful. Those who said they ate soy foods listed tofu and soy burgers as the ones they ate most frequently.

According to the FDA, studies have shown that soy protein, when part of a diet low in saturated fat and cholesterol, can reduce the risk of coronary heart disease. Foods containing at least 6.25 grams of soy protein per serving can carry labels claiming a heart health benefit. Soy protein differs from other vegetable proteins because it changes how the liver processes cholesterol. To gain heart health benefits, you need to eat at least 25 grams of soy protein a day.

Soy protein comes from soybeans, one of the major sources of protein worldwide. Soy may be added to many different types of foods and beverages. It is used to make tofu, some types of noodles, and meat substitutes such as soy burgers. Soy milk is frequently prescribed for babies allergic to other types of milk.

Sweet Potatoes, Please

These roots of gold deserve more attention. The sweet potato is the richest vegetable source of vitamin A and is loaded with beta-carotene; sweet potatoes and yams are one of the few good sources of vitamin E that are not loaded with fat.

Time for Tea?

Tea drinking originated in China nearly five thousand years ago and spread throughout Asia and the world, becoming firmly entrenched in the diet and lifestyles of many cultures. After water, tea is the second most consumed beverage worldwide. Tea has long been held in high esteem for its soothing and medicinal qualities. New scientific evidence suggests that drinking tea may reduce the risk of heart disease and cancer, lower blood pressure, and even help prevent tooth decay. Researchers at Kyushu University in Japan have identified four components in tea that help mop up bacteria in your mouth that promote tooth decay. Tannin, catechin, caffeine, and tocopherol in tea help increase the acid resistance of tooth enamel.

It takes just three minutes of brewing for tea to release its health-promoting compounds. Tea is high in polyphenols—a type of antioxidant—and may be beneficial in reducing cancer risk. Polyphenols in tea make up 30 percent of tea's dry weight. In fact, tea bags are better than large loose tea leaves because the tiny pulverized leaves provide greater surface area in contact with hot water and can release more polyphenols.

Differences among the three types of tea—green, black, and oolong—result from the degree of processing and the level of contact with oxygen. Green tea is not exposed to oxygen, and after processing most closely resembles the chemical composition of the fresh tea leaf. Perhaps that's why green tea seems to confer the most beneficial health effects. Black tea is exposed to the air for up to three hours. Oolong tea has a shorter period of oxidation, and falls between green and black tea in health benefits.

Selected Studies

- The antioxidant activity of twenty-two common vegetables and green and black tea were measured. Investigators found that green and black tea were much more effective antioxidants against a common free radical than all of the vegetables tested, including broccoli, carrots, and garlic (*Journal of Agricultural and Food Chemistry,* December 1996).

- Drinking at least one cup of tea daily could reduce the risk of heart attack by 44 percent, according to research presented at the Society of Medicine Conference in London in July 1999. This study used black tea and found no differences if you drank it hot or cold or added milk, sugar, or lemon.

Tomatoes Catch Up

For centuries tomatoes were thought to be toxic, capable of causing everything from appendicitis to cancer to mental illness. Today tomatoes are one of America's favorite foods. We eat more tomatoes, both fresh and processed, than nearly any other fruit or vegetable. That's good news because tomatoes contain the red pigment lycopene, a fantastic phytochemical. Lycopene can withstand exposure to high heat, so canned tomatoes and tomato sauce are rich sources. If you cook your fresh tomatoes just a bit, it causes the cell walls to burst and even more lycopene is released for your body to absorb.

Did you know that salsa has replaced catsup as the most consumed condiment in the United States? That's good news because it's easy to down a serving or two of tomatoes in the form of salsa.

Vegetables: Can It

Fresh is best when it comes to choosing vegetables, right? Not necessarily, according to research from the human nutrition researchers at the University of Illinois. Processed vegetables lose some vitamin C when heated, but it is almost exactly the same amount that fresh vegetables lose when they're cooked. Most fresh vegetables are picked several weeks before they arrive at your local produce counter. Nutrient losses during shipping and storage can be equal to or greater than what is lost during cooking. The nutritional value of fresh produce decreases with time. According to the University of Minnesota Extension Service, nearly half of some vitamins may be lost within a few day of harvesting unless fresh produce is quickly cooled or preserved. Within one to two weeks, even refrigerated produce will continue to lose up to half or more of some vitamins.

Food companies choose top-quality varieties of produce for processing—top quality means high in nutrients. Varieties grown for canning and freezing start out with more vitamins and minerals than the typical fresh produce shipped to your local supermarket. If you're going to cook your vegetables, it doesn't matter much which form you choose—fresh, frozen, or canned; just eat them. Choose raw vegetables from local sources when possible. If you're cutting back on sodium, choose fresh and plain varieties of frozen vegetables. You can also drain canned vegetables, but you'll be pouring off some beneficial nutrients along with the extra sodium.

NUTRITION ACTION If you're serious about not wasting nutrients, start storing leftover liquid from canned vegetables. Keep a pitcher in your freezer to collect the broth. Keep adding new broth on top of the frozen portion until you have enough to use as soup stock. Simply thaw and use this nutrient gold mine the next time you make soup. If sodium is a concern, buy low-sodium canned vegetables.

Wine: Health Aid or Health Hazard?

Wine drinkers have a lower risk of developing certain cancers than people who consume equal amounts of beer or hard liquor. Breast cancer isn't one of those, however. Daily wine consumption may actually increase your risk for cancer of the breast. Alcoholic drinks have carcinogenic properties that increase the odds of getting cancer of the upper digestive tract, but grapes (especially red grapes) have a substance called reversatrol that counteracts the damaging effect. As few as 1 to 4 glasses of wine a month can reduce the risk for macular degeneration (loss of central vision) by 20 percent.

Selected Studies

Dr. Morten Gronbaek and colleagues at the Institute of Preventive Medicine in Copenhagen studied more than 28,000 men and women over thirteen years to determine the relationship between types of alcoholic drinks and cancer in the upper digestive tract. They found that people who drank only beer and hard liquor had a higher risk of getting cancer than nondrinkers or those who drank only wine (*British Journal of Medicine,* September 1998). Wine should be your drink of choice if you choose alcoholic beverages—in moderation, of course.

Zucchini: What a Squash!

Dark-skinned zucchini, like its squash and pumpkin relatives, provides the antioxidant beta-carotene. The edible yellow-orange blossoms contain vitamin C and potassium, too. Zucchini is perhaps best known for its versatility—you can put it in anything from soups and salads to breads, muffins, and pancakes. Don't peel your zucchini, since the skin is where the bulk of its nutrients are found.

THE BAD NEWS: NUTRIENT THIEVES

Nutrients are always team players; they all work together. Optimal intakes of all vitamins, minerals, and other essential nutrients are the foundation of good nutrition. But even if you eat right, there are nutrient thieves just waiting to rob you of those precious goods and compromise your health. Here's a quick list of some of the most common nutrient busters, with more detail on a few to follow.

- *Alcohol* destroys a variety of nutrients it comes in contact with, even though it may offer other health benefits.
- *Antacids* can deplete your stores of vitamin D (though some add calcium).

- *Caffeine* overload speeds up metabolism and pumps vitamins and minerals through your system too fast for optimal absorption.
- *Cooking* with high temperatures, rough food handling, cutting and chopping food, and cooking foods in lots of water can all speed up nutrient losses.
- *Diuretics* pull water and water-soluble vitamins out in urine. You can also lose electrolytes such as potassium and magnesium.
- *Excess fiber* isn't recommended for the very young and very old. They lose B vitamins and some minerals that can't be absorbed with too much fiber present.
- *Oil-based laxatives* can leach vitamins A, D, E, and K from your gut. Overuse of any laxative can speed how fast food moves through your system, and that limits nutrient absorption.
- *Pollution* from smog, car exhaust, and chemical run-off into water increases free radicals in your system. Free radicals speed up cell damage.
- *Smoking* increases free radical action, and that raises your need for vitamin C; but don't take supplements because too much vitamin C increases the nicotine output in your urine, and that will increase how much nicotine you need to satisfy your addiction. Eat more citrus fruits and juices and other foods high in vitamin C.
- *Stress* increases free radical activity in your system.

Alcohol Effects

Alcohol consumption is an important issue to consider. Alcohol has a tremendous ability to eat away at both your nutritional and overall health. A social drinker who weighs 150 pounds and has normal liver function metabolizes 7 to 14 grams of alcohol (6 to 12 ounces of beer) in one hour. If you drink slightly less than the amount of alcohol your liver can metabolize, your blood alcohol content will remain low. When the rate of alcohol exceeds your liver's metabolic capacity, your blood alcohol will rise and symptoms of intoxication appear.

Women cannot metabolize as much alcohol as men because their stomachs have lower levels of a key alcohol-metabolizing enzyme, alcohol dehydrogenase. Women also are much quicker to develop alcohol-related health problems, such as cirrhosis of the liver, than men with the same drinking history. Alcohol is toxic to the cells that line both the esophagus and the stomach, and heavy drinking increases the risk of cancer at these sites. Large quantities of alcohol can lead to high blood pressure and scar tissue formation in the heart muscle. This can lead to fat infiltration into the heart muscle and cause an enlarged heart.

Moderate alcohol consumption, on the other hand, may have some beneficial effects. "Moderate" is defined by the U.S. Dietary Guidelines as no more than one drink per day for women and two drinks per day for men. And no, you can't save them up and have a six-pack while watching the game on Sunday and still be a moderate drinker. A variety of research shows that a small amount of alcohol daily can have the beneficial effect of lowering the risk for heart disease. Many frail elderly find that a small alcoholic drink before dinner may help stimulate their appetite. That also works for others, too, so if you're trying to lose weight, remember that alcohol before meals will make you want to eat more. As with all things, alcohol—if you choose to drink—in moderation is okay.

Go Figure
1 drink of alcohol = 4 oz. of wine, 12 oz. of beer, or 1½ oz. of hard liquor

Caffeine: Trouble Brewing?

It's America's favorite drug. Caffeine is a mild stimulant that can fight fatigue, improve your mood, and even boost mental and physical performance. Studies have shown that as little as 32 mg of caffeine—the amount in ⅓ cup of coffee—helps people pay better attention to a long, repetitious series of tones or pictures. It's true that caffeine can enhance how you perform monotonous tasks like keyboarding, listening to a boring speaker, or prolonged driving. Too much caffeine over time, though, is addictive. If you want to cut back, do it gradually to help prevent mood swings and irritability.

For years, researchers have tried to get a handle on caffeine's relationship to chronic disease. No strong positive association has ever been proven because it's hard to look at just caffeine intake. For example, many heavy coffee drinkers also smoke, consume lots of alcohol, and tend to have high-fat diets. Coffee has also changed over time. Odds are you're not familiar with cafestol and kahweol. They are two substances found in the oils of coffee grounds. As long as you drink instant coffee or use a drip filter (as do most home coffeemakers), you won't be exposed to this twosome that's believed to raise LDL (bad) cholesterol and triglycerides. Some researchers think that the popularity of drip coffeemakers since 1975 (instead of perked or brewed coffee) explains why more recent studies show no higher risk of heart disease in coffee drinkers. Since caffeine is a drug usually found in foods and beverages with little redeeming nutrient value, it makes sense to limit your consumption.

Caffeine in Common Foods and Medications

	Average Caffeine (mg)
Coffee	
Espresso, 2 oz.	120
Regular, brewed 6 oz.	105
Instant, 6 oz.	55
Tea	
Black, 6 oz.	36
Oolong, 6 oz.	35
Green, 6 oz.	30
Soft Drinks	
Surge 12 oz.	72
Mountain Dew 12 oz.	55
Coke, varieties 12 oz.	35–50
Sunkist Orange 12 oz.	42
Pepsi 12 oz.	38
Chocolate	
Unsweetened baking chocolate, 1 oz.	58
Milk chocolate candy bar, 1.5-oz. average	11
Pain Relievers	
Aspirin-Free Excedrin, Excedrin Extra Strength, 1 caplet	65
Vanquish, 1 caplet	33
Stimulants	
No Doz Maximum Strength 1 caplet	200
Vivarin, 1 tablet or 1 caplet	200

Source: Manufacturers' data

Fake Foods

Foods without fat or calories that taste great—that's what the American consumer seems to want. According to a 1996 survey done by the Calorie Control Council, 88 percent of adults said they consume low-fat, reduced-fat, or fat-free foods and beverages. But fat substitutes and reduced-fat foods do not make up for poor eating habits.

Sugar and fat substitutes have failed miserably. They were supposed to let us have our cake and eat it, too. That's the problem. We want to drink a diet pop with a chocolate candy bar. With fat-free cookies, the whole package sometimes becomes one serving instead of two or three cookies. Don't fool yourself; these "substitutes" usually aren't substituting for anything.

PART II

Getting What You Need

4

Eating Style Options

In this section we will look at age-related differences that affect nutritional needs. We'll also compare and contrast a variety of eating styles from around the world and across the centuries. Almost any system of food choices can be adapted to provide optimal nutrition for your own individual needs. The challenge is in learning enough about a particular system to understand the subtleties. Food and food choices are deeply rooted in cultural systems. Within a given culture, values and food choices seem reasonable and make sense in that context. What seems to be logical, sensible, important, and reasonable in one culture may seem dumb, irrational, or unimportant to an outsider. For these reasons, be cautious about making moral judgments on alternative eating styles.

Throughout life, people everywhere need the same nutrients, though in different amounts at different times. Some health concerns are lifelong, and others are particularly important at specific stages of life. For example, we know that coronary heart disease develops slowly over time and learning healthful eating habits in childhood can decrease risk as an adult. Teens and pregnant women need extra amounts of particular nutrients, including calcium and calories, to foster the extra growth their bodies require.

IT'S A SMALL, SMALL WORLD

Children are not miniature adults. What may be the ideal food choices for you are probably not right for young children. Obviously kids don't need the same quantity of food as adults. Quality of food should also be a consideration. Many cultures do have specific recommendations for feeding children. There is no doubt that growing bodies and minds have unique dietary needs, particularly for energy, fat, and calcium.

Make Mealtime Quality Time

According to research from Cincinnati Children's Hospital Medical Centers, families that eat meals together have better-adjusted teens. Children who ate with their families at least five times a week were less likely to use drugs or become depressed compared to those who ate with parents just three times a week. It's also an opportunity for adults to act as role models and display healthful eating habits. Children often imitate what their parents do, but not always what they say. If you don't eat your vegetables, don't expect your children to. Look at it this way: having a baby is one of the best motivators for improving your own nutrition. You finally have to practice what you preach!

Eating with others promotes positive connections. It's a pattern that should start as soon as infants are able to eat solid foods. Mealtime is a primary setting for developing social skills and awareness. Preschoolers gain a sense of manners and consideration for others by passing foods and not taking second helpings until everyone has been served. These eating and social skills can transfer to other everyday activities. Not learning these skills can have serious consequences.

Eating meals together is often the only opportunity for parents and children to stay in tune with each other. Schedule conflicts can make that a challenge. To get back into the habit of family meals:

- Establish fun traditions, for example, Sunday brunch.
- Look beyond dinner: Breakfast, weekend lunches, and snack time count, too.
- Assign everyone a role in getting family meals on the table.

INK UP to http://www.kidsfood.com for fun sites for kids to explore foods and nutrition on their own.

Teen Eating Machines

Adolescence is a time of turbulent changes, both psychological and physical. A variety of hormones trigger four major physical changes:

> growth rate increases
>
> height and weight increase
>
> body composition changes
>
> sexual maturity is achieved

There is a wide variation in growth rate from teenager to teenager. Most girls begin their growth spurt two or more years before boys their same age. Girls gain proportionately more fat than boys, so that by age 20 they have about twice as much body fat as males.

Needs for almost every nutrient increase during these years of tremendous growth. Girls need more nutrients at a younger age to support optimal growth and development. Boys need more nutrients and calories and continue to need more food as adults to maintain their larger muscle mass.

Like many adults, teens tend to consume iron, calcium, magnesium, vitamin A, and vitamin B_6 at levels that fall short of their needs for these nutrients.

NUTRITION ACTIONS FOR FEEDING TEENS
You don't have control over everything teenagers eat, but you can indirectly influence what they eat at home. Here are some ideas to help teens develop healthful food habits.
- Provide quick-to-fix breakfast foods such as cereal, muffins, bagels, yogurt, or leftovers from last night's dinner (macaroni and cheese, pizza, etc.).
- If your teen skips breakfast or isn't hungry, offer foods for the backpack to be eaten later (fresh fruit, canned fruit or vegetable juices, a sandwich, etc.).
- Anticipate when your teen will be hungry and stock the refrigerator with nutritious snack foods.
- Teach teens to cook so they have the basic skills for kitchen independence.
- Arrange mealtimes that don't conflict with activities important to your teen.

OLDER ADULTS

Age has it privileges—and its aches and pains. However, symptoms once attributed to "old age" are often the result of poor eating habits. Beginning at age 30, flavor and aroma perceptions begin to decline. At age 70 these decreases become more noticeable, and they decline significantly at age 80. In fact, people over 60 may need two to eight times higher concentrations of salt or sugar to achieve the same taste sensations as a young adult. These sensory losses are not just part of normal aging, but also develop from diseases and certain medications that alter taste and smell.

Ready for some more bad news? Somewhere between the ages of 40 and 50 your calorie needs decrease by up to 10 percent every ten years. That translates into about 100 calories less per day per decade. Yet you still need almost every key nutrient in the same amounts as younger people, and there are some essential nutrients whose requirements actually increase with age (vitamins B_6, B_{12}, D, E, and the minerals chromium and zinc). These nutrients aid in digestion, nutrient absorption, nerve functioning, help to balance blood sugar levels, and strengthen your immune system.

How to Eat Well When You're Not Motivated
- Plan to eat with a friend as often as possible—even cook and shop together. Eating with others often improves your appetite.
- Buy precut fruits, vegetables, and prepared salads to keep on hand when you don't feel like washing and chopping.
- Enhance the aroma of foods by adding peppers, garlic, onions, lemon, or mint.

- Use herb blends and spices to add more flavor to bland foods. The nerve that carries herb and spice sensations seems to be less affected by aging than other flavor-carrying nerves.
- At mealtimes, eat the most nutritious foods first, when you are hungrier.
- Chew your food well. The longer food is in your mouth and mixing with saliva, the more time your taste buds have to send those flavor sensations to your brain.
- Alternate bites of different foods on your plate. Your taste buds can get "tired" of one food, and the flavor intensity decreases if you eat one thing at a time.
- If you seem to "fill up" after just a few bites, try eating six smaller meals rather than three large ones.

DIETARY GUIDELINES: A WORLDVIEW

If you want to be healthy, eat like a healthy person. But which healthy person should you imitate? Nutrition needs to be personalized for your unique circumstances. One starting point to consider is your ethnic heritage. As much as we have in common as human beings, there are also subtle variations that make each of us unique. If we all have very similar heart and circulatory systems, then why are some groups of people more prone to heart disease or high blood pressure? Many people intolerant to milk never develop osteoporosis, even though they don't get nearly the recommended amount of calcium. Part of this mystery can be explained by natural adaptation.

Girth of a Nation

Compare the average weight of both men and women (based on a height of 5'4") from around the world. These dramatic differences may be even more profound today, since the data for this study was collected more than a decade ago.

Country or Region	Weight in Pounds*
United States of America	160
Southern Europe	152
Eastern Europe	151
Western and Central Europe	145
Northern Europe	145
South and Central America	141
Africa	136
Asia	123

* Combined average weights of men and women.
Source: Adapted from INTERSALT data from *Obesity,* 1992

Think about the first time you sat face to face with a computer. Many people were resistant to this new technology. It was difficult to use, you didn't understand how it worked, and it took a lot of practice to get things right. Once you had some training, actually read the instruction manual, or pleaded with someone to show you what to do, things clicked. This same process is important for understanding eating patterns from around the world. For example, here's a country-by-country snapshot of nutrition issues deemed important for good health. Most North American, Asian, and European countries have used dietary guidelines for many years. As rates of obesity and chronic disease increase in developing countries, they too are adopting national nutrition guidelines. These recommendations take into account varying nutritional priorities, food supplies, and cultural eating patterns of each country. Obviously there will be differences and similarities. Most important is what they have in common. Worldwide consensus shows that all people should:

- Eat a variety of foods.
- Maintain a healthy weight and active lifestyle.
- Eat a diet low in fat, especially saturated fat.
- Limit sodium and sugar.
- Avoid alcohol, or drink in moderation.

Cultural Diversity in Dietary Guidelines

Here's a quick view of dietary guidelines from around the world, highlighting each country's unique aspects.

Australia has a special guideline to encourage and support breast-feeding. Special guidelines for children and teens stress that low-fat diets are not appropriate for young children. Aussie children are encouraged to drink water when they are thirsty.

Canada recommends no more than 5 percent of total calories be alcohol, or two drinks daily, whichever is less. Caffeine consumption should be kept to the equivalent of four or fewer cups of coffee daily. Fluoridation of all community water supplies is a national priority.

Denmark has just a few guidelines—short and to the point. Don't eat too much. Eat coarse foods. Eat more bread, corn, potatoes, vegetables, and fruit. Eat less fat, fatty meats, whole-milk dairy products, and sugar.

France wants its citizens to eat three meals a day and eat more vegetable proteins.

Germany promotes eating small meals more often to help people keep calories under control. German nutritionists also advise to prepare foods safely.

Canada's Food Guide to Healthy Living

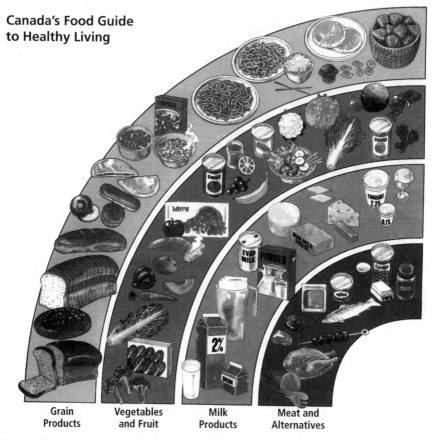

| Grain Products | Vegetables and Fruit | Milk Products | Meat and Alternatives |

Source: Minister of Supply and Services, Canada, 1992.

Hungary gets specific on milk consumption and suggests drinking half a liter (about 2 cups) of low-fat milk daily. Four or five meals a day is recommended for hungry Hungarians, but none too rich or too light. Alcohol is forbidden for children and pregnant women.

Israel wins for the best graphic description of its dietary guidelines. It prefers a figure-eight-shaped cup or chalice filled with fruits and vegetables and topped off with water. A belt cinches in the waist or stem of the glass and represents a small fat intake. Grains are the large bottom portion of the cup.

Japan is the only country to take a stab at defining variety. Eat thirty foodstuffs a day and eat staples, main dishes, and side dishes together. Its sodium limit of 10,000 mg a day is more than four times higher than the U.S. sodium guidelines. The Japanese could inspire the world with their final guideline: Happy eating makes for happy family life; sit down and eat together and talk; treasure favorite family foods and home cooking.

Korea is the only country to mention taking good care of your teeth as an important part of nutrition. The recommended fat intake of 20 percent of calories is the lowest in the world. Koreans also take a philosophical approach to eating: Keep harmony between diet and daily life and enjoy meals.

The Netherlands' nutrition policymakers prefer a technically precise position. Percentages and target intakes of nutrients abound. The sodium guideline is 8,000 mg a day. One guideline is the caution to realize that current alcohol consumption is far too high in many cases.

New Zealand's basic guidelines are short and to the point. What they lack in length, they make up for by including six additional sets of guidelines. Infants and toddlers, children, teens, older people, pregnant women, and breast-feeding women each have individualized standard recommendations.

Norway's National Nutrition Council has a great motto: Food plus Joy equals Health.

The Philippines proclaims basic guidelines with no frills. Eat clean and safe food, practice a healthful lifestyle, and promote breast-feeding and proper weaning.

South Africa is the most recent country to adopt nutrition guidelines. Because there is a transition from rural, traditional eating patterns to a more Western lifestyle, it's understandable that the recommendations mimic those of most industrialized countries. One notable exception is the recommendation to drink lots of clean, safe water. South Africa is also working on adapting guidelines for children under 5 and people with special dietary needs.

Thailand's guidelines almost mimic U.S. recommendations. They do suggest that the people of Thailand recognize and eat well-prepared food that is free of microorganisms and food contaminants. From the Japanese they have borrowed the motto: A happy family is when family members eat together and enjoy treasured family recipes and good home cooking.

The United Kingdom's National Food Guide uses a plate of food rather than a pyramid for its graphic. It resembles a divided plate similar to a school lunch tray. One-third contains fruits and vegetables, one-third is grains, and the final third includes dairy products and meat, fish, and alternatives. Fats and sweets are given just a sliver of the last section of the plate.

The United States has not yet integrated the science and social aspects of nutrition into its guidelines. No "enjoy your meals" or "treasure family foods" mottoes for us. We don't even encourage breast-feeding our babies.

Food Guide Pyramid:
A Guide to Daily Food Choices

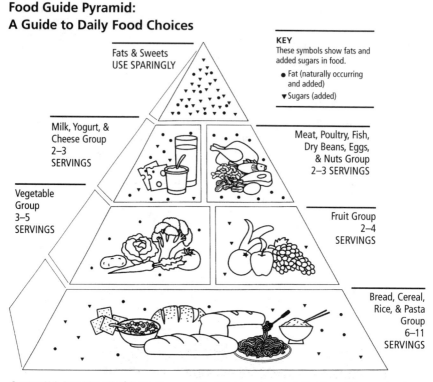

KEY
These symbols show fats and added sugars in food.

● Fat (naturally occurring and added)
▼ Sugars (added)

Fats & Sweets
USE SPARINGLY

Milk, Yogurt, & Cheese Group
2–3 SERVINGS

Meat, Poultry, Fish, Dry Beans, Eggs, & Nuts Group
2–3 SERVINGS

Vegetable Group
3–5 SERVINGS

Fruit Group
2–4 SERVINGS

Bread, Cereal, Rice, & Pasta Group
6–11 SERVINGS

Source: U.S. Department of Agriculture and the U.S. Department of Health and Human Services

Water is still a forgotten nutrient in the United States. Remember that dietary guidelines apply to your total way of eating, not just one food, one meal, or even one day. It's your food choices over time that impact your health.

The Challenge of Nutrition Guidelines

Archaeologists and historians have unearthed details of how our ancient ancestors foraged, hunted, and harvested food. It is clear that regional weather patterns have had a major influence on staple foods worldwide. For example, tropical regions with abundant rainfall are ideally suited for growth of fruits, which are prominent in the diets of local people. Cereal grains are another example. Rice is a staple in Southeast Asia because the climate is ideally suited for its growth. South America's staple grain is corn. In North America, wheat grows well and is widely consumed. The extremely rugged terrain of many Nordic countries and their proximity to the sea results in a strong reliance on the ocean for food.

Importing and exporting of foods worldwide has transformed and expanded the variety of foods available to many people. This unprecedented year-round availability of so many foods should have led to major

The Tumbling Pyramid: How Americans Really Eat

This tumbling pyramid is closer to reality than the recommended (and balanced) food guide pyramid. The lesson: most of us need to eat more from the middle of the pyramid and trim back on the fats, oils, and sweets.

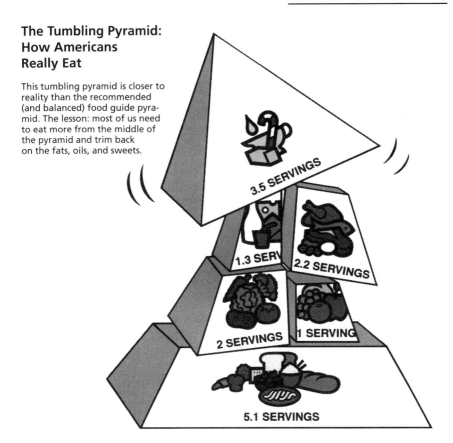

3.5 SERVINGS

1.3 SERV

2.2 SERVINGS

2 SERVINGS   1 SERVING

5.1 SERVINGS

Source: *Eating in America Today, Edition II: A Dietary Pattern and Intake Report*

health improvements worldwide. And it has. People today are (on the whole) taller and stronger, and live longer than their ancestors. World food trade has also hastened the spread of poor eating habits to cultures and countries that can least afford them. It's great to be able to bring home fresh berries and bananas from the grocery store in the midst of a Midwest blizzard. But it's a shame—and dangerous—that soft drinks and empty-calorie snack foods are for sale in poverty-stricken Third World countries.

It's important to understand that changing your eating style might fend off heart disease or cancer. It's quite another step to do something about it. Food is more than just something to eat. Food choices and eating styles reflect wide-ranging cultural, social, and psychological factors.

Traditional American food patterns are changing in a number of ways. More women are working. We increasingly rely on food technology. Household size is smaller and more people live alone. Fewer people have time to cook or prepare meals. The average time spent in meal preparation today is less than 15 minutes for dinner. Compare that to over an hour just fifteen years ago. Even the definition of cooking has changed. Cooking today is defined by actually touching food with your hands when you prepare it. Heating a frozen dinner isn't considered cooking, but opening a prepared bagged salad and mixing in croutons and cheese is! A lot of meal preparation in the United States is really meal assembly. You divide up a packaged tossed salad mix, microwave a frozen entree, open a package of dinner rolls, and yell "dinner's ready." Often it's children and teens, not the adults, who assume the main role in choosing and preparing meals.

Packaged cake mixes were one of the first convenience items that consumers liked. Just crack an egg or two, add some milk or water, and you had a "homemade" cake. Major food companies were so delighted with sales they invented new and improved cake mixes. All you had to add was water. Sales nose-dived and the new mixes were taken off the market. Why? If you didn't get to crack an egg, it didn't feel like cooking.

Obsessed Eating

There are additional concerns, beyond meeting basic nutritional goals. The incidence rate for eating disorder diseases, especially among young women and girls, is soaring. Self-induced anorexia (severe undereating) and bulimia (compulsive overeating, then purging) are psychological and physical disorders found only in highly developed countries with a preoccupation for thinness. Bulimia and anorexia share similarities even though each is a different disorder. Both are defined by an intense preoccupation with food and body weight, and can be life-threatening. Now a third type of disordered eating has been identified.

Orthorexia (or-tho-REX-ee-ah) is the newest eating disorder to add to the list of modern ailments. Orthorexia is a psychological obsession that results in the systematic elimination of specific foods or entire food groups believed to be harmful to one's health. "Whereas anorexics or bulimics focus on the quantity of food, orthorexics fixate on quality," says Dr. Steve Bratman, a Colorado physician who coined this new term in 1997. Orthorexics fool themselves into believing they have to eat the way they do. They think their strict control over food prevents cravings, fatigue, and a whole host of other symptoms. Women are far more likely to fall into this trap than men. Obsession over food is a way of life for many women. Here are some common examples of crossing the line between disciplined dieter and eating extremist:

Allergy Activists spend hours at the grocery store and on the phone to food manufacturers asking questions about foods and food additives they think cause allergic reactions. These people have never seen an allergist or had any testing done to verify the presence of true food allergies. Be careful not to confuse these folks with people who have true food allergies. The main difference is that allergy activists are usually "allergic" to foods that can't possibly cause allergic reactions.

Fat Phobics are experts at detecting the slightest trace of fat in a food. Their goal is a no-fat diet. Such a diet is not only an impossibility, it is also unhealthful.

Sugar Sleuths scour food labels for any trace of sugar. Although most sugar is an empty-calorie food, there are naturally occurring sugars in nutritious foods like fruit, juice, and milk products.

EATING STYLES

A healthful way of eating can take many forms. No one food provides all the nutrients required for optimal health. Foods can be combined in many different ways to make up a lifestyle approach that provides all the nutrients you need. As you evaluate the different eating styles and philosophies summarized here, use the following questions as a guide to help you determine if they are right for you:

- Are a variety of nutritious foods from every nutrient category included?
- Are foods eaten in balanced amounts?
- Are recommended fat, sugar, and sodium levels modest?
- Will this way of eating fit my lifestyle?
- Will the foods be easy to find and prepare?

Ayurvedic

This five thousand–year–old system of medicine from India is the oldest recorded healing therapy still in existence today. Ayurveda (ah-yoor-VAY-dah) is a Sanskrit word that means "the science or knowledge of life." As such it embraces every aspect of who you are and what you do. An Ayurvedic doctor will tell you what your dosha (body/personality) type is and then customize a plan of foods, herbs, exercise, and other lifestyle habits that will produce health and harmony for you. Ayurveda is based on an immense system of classifications.

Ayurveda emphasizes oneness with nature, longevity, and enlightenment and has a strong nutritional component. In Ayurveda, the physical body is believed to be made of the same elements found in nature: *akash* (space), *vayu* (air), *tejas* (fire), *jala* (water), and *prithvi* (earth). These elements are further organized into a combination of three different humors or personalities. These body humors include *kapha* (calm, steady, good-natured), *vata* (spiritual and creative), and *pitta* (impulsive and strong-willed). Ayurveda also classifies foods and medicinal herbs into six major tastes—sweet, salty, sour, pungent, astringent, and bitter—and six major qualities—oily, heavy, light, dry, hot, and cold. Climate and age are also factored into your dietary regimen. It's impossible to explain such a complex system in a few pages. Use this chart for a simplistic overview of the combinations.

Ayurvedic Combinations

Style	Climate	Age	Meal Frequency	Foods	Tastes	Avoid	Special Added Nutrients
Anti-Vata	cold, dry, windy climates such as high deserts or high plains	old age	frequent regular meals	warm, heavy, moistening, strengthening	sweet, sour, salty	fast, instant, and junk foods, beans	vitamin A, D, E, C, zinc, and calcium
Anti-Pitta	hot tropical or desert climates such as the U.S. South	middle age	three meals a day, don't eat late dinner	cool, slightly dry, a little heavy	sweet, bitter, astringent	mild foods, alcohol, nuts, oil, spices, animal products	vitamins B and K, calcium, and iron
Anti-Kapha	damp, cold regions like the U.S. Midwest Northeast, and Northwest	youth and childhood	3 meals a day, but eat less in morning and evening, avoid breakfast	warm, light, dry	pungent, bitter, astringent	Oils, dairy foods, animal products, sweeteners	spices, herbs, and enzymes instead of vitamins and minerals except vitamin B

Tastes and qualities have more to do with how a food affects the body than with its actual flavor and texture. For example, milk is considered sweet, oily, heavy, and cold, while spinach is astringent, light, and hot. A proper Ayurvedic meal includes a variety of foods representing different tastes and qualities. It is essential that the correct method of preparation is used, amounts of food are appropriate, and the emotional attitude of both the food preparer and eater are harmonious. As a health system, Ayurveda attempts to use good nutrition, along with many other lifestyle approaches, to bring the body into balance and maintain it there. This approach is based on the belief that improper diet is the cause of most disease.

Homeopathy

Homeopathy is a relative newcomer, dating back to the late 1700s when Samuel Hahnemann, a German physician, began this new system of care. At the time, homeopathy was a welcome change from bloodletting, leeching, purging, and other medical procedures of the day. The word *homeopathy* means "like treats like." It's based on giving minute amounts of substances that would cause the very disease you're trying to cure. Treatment with such small doses is believed to stimulate your own natural defense system and encourage self-healing. The doses used are so small they are unlikely to have any bad effects, but there's no proof they help either. Homeopathy seeks to take advantage of your natural healing power. The complete range of symptoms is considered: emotions, brain, and body.

Homeopotists are the first to admit that they can't explain the mechanism that makes homeopathic medicine work. It's difficult to discuss homeopathy objectively. The bases of this medical practice are very thin and routinely exaggerated. Only scanty scientific evidence is available to prove that homeopathy has any health benefits. Because homeopathic remedies were actually less dangerous than those used earlier, many medical practitioners adopted them. At the turn of the twentieth century, popularity declined. There is no specific diet or set of nutritional recommendations used in homeopathy. If you are diagnosed with a particular problem, part of the healing antidote prescribed for you may come with diet restrictions to avoid certain foods or food ingredients. For example, you might be told to avoid coffee or all caffeine-containing products.

Macrobiotics

The original macrobiotic diet was developed by Yukikazu Sakurazawa in 1913. This self-taught Japanese pioneer believed that an ideal food plan was based on grains and the Asian system of balance, yin and yang. Meat, eggs, dairy products, sugar, caffeine, alcohol, and processed foods were forbidden. Sakurazawa's favorite student, Michio Kushi, brought macrobiotics to America "as a healing response to the devastation of World War II." Today, Kushi and his wife, Aveline, run the Kushi Institute in Becket, Massachusetts, where they work with practitioners and individuals to teach their updated macrobiotic system of eating. Kushi's macrobiotics is different from the "hippie" Zen macrobiotic of the 1960s (which was a severe diet that claimed brown rice was the perfect—and therefore the only—food to eat).

Kushi's Macrobiotic Eating Plan

Food Group	Proportion of Diet	Varieties
Whole grains	50–60%	barley, buckwheat, millet, oats, rice, and wheat
		noodles: ramen, saifun, soba, somen, udon
Vegetables	20–25%	bok choy, burdock, collard greens, daikon, kale, lotus root, watercress
Seaweed and beans	5–10%	seaweeds: arame, dulse, hiziki, kombu, nori, wakame
		beans: adzuki, natto, soybeans, tempeh, tofu
Soups	5–10%	miso

Note: If you live in a very cold climate, some white-flesh fish is included; if you live in a tropical climate, some fruits are allowed.

If you choose a macrobiotic eating style, here's what you need to know:

You'll feel worse before you feel better. Common adjustment symptoms include fatigue, mild aches and pains, fever, chills, coughing, perspiration, frequent urination, skin discharges, skin rashes, unusual body odor, diarrhea and/or constipation, reduction in sexual desire, irritability, and temporary loss of menstrual cycle in women. Advocates suggest these effects happen because your body is purging toxins. Once you've gotten rid of them, you'll supposedly feel better. However, not everyone does.

You will need to eat a wide variety of foods. Permitted foods are so limited in macrobiotics that it is essential to eat a little of practically everything that is allowed. That's the best way to ensure you get as many nutrients from food as possible.

You should take supplements. Even though supplements are not advised, it's practically impossible to get enough B_{12} from the allowed foods. Better yet would be a complete multivitamin-mineral supplement. Be sure it includes vitamin C, vitamin E, calcium, magnesium, and iron.

This diet is not for kids. A population study in the Netherlands found that children under 2 fed macrobiotic diets had retarded growth, fat and muscle loss, and slow motor development. Pregnant women may also risk the health of their developing baby if their nutrient levels fall too low.

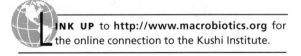
INK UP to http://www.macrobiotics.org for the online connection to the Kushi Institute.

Mediterranean Diet

During World War II, heart disease rates plummeted in countries with shortages of meat and dairy products. When world-renowned researcher Dr. Ancel Keys and his wife traveled around Europe and Africa in the 1950s measuring blood cholesterol levels, they noticed that affluent people, who were eating more meat and dairy, were more likely to have high cholesterol and suffer heart attacks than poor people. Keys assembled a research team that looked at the diets, lifestyles, and blood cholesterol levels of more than 12,000 healthy middle-age men in Finland, Greece, Italy, Japan, the Netherlands, the United States, and Yugoslavia. The participants in the Seven Countries Study ranged from 2,000 U.S. and 750 Italian railroad workers to 500 faculty members of the University of Belgrade to 1,000 residents of two fishing villages in Japan.

After five, ten, fifteen, and twenty years, Keys counted how many people had—or had died of—heart disease. After ten years, the 775 men from Finland fared the worst: 28 percent had developed heart disease. The Finns were eating more saturated fat (mostly from cheese and butter) than almost anyone else—24 percent of their calories. That's double what Americans now eat. The Japanese residents of the fishing villages of Tanushimaru and Ushibuka ate the least fat (9 percent of calories) and saturated fat (3 percent of calories). Only 5 percent of them had developed heart disease. That was far better than the Finns, but it wasn't the best. That honor went to the 655 men from the Greek island of Crete. After ten years, 2 percent of them had developed heart disease, and none of them had died. Amazingly, the Greeks were eating about as much total fat as the artery-clogged Finns. Their intake of saturated fat was far lower (about 8 percent of calories), but it wasn't as low as that of the mostly rice-and-vegetable Japanese diet.

The Mediterranean diet, back in the 1950s and 1960s, was dominated by olive oil and whole-grain bread. These two foods alone accounted for 50 to over 60 percent of total calories. The diet was also rich in beans, fresh fruits, and vegetables. Meat, sugar, and most dairy products were consumed in very small amounts. It's also important to keep in mind that the lifestyle and physical activity patterns in this culture decades ago were vastly different than U.S. lifestyles are today.

If you are slim and have low HDL cholesterol, a diet rich in monounsaturated fat (like olive oil) may protect your heart. But if you have a tendency to gain weight, a diet rich in monounsaturated fat may make you fatter, which can raise your risk of heart and other diseases. Olive oil is rich in monounsaturated fat, "which appears to raise blood levels of HDL" (the good cholesterol), explains researcher Scott Grundy of the University of Texas Health Sciences Center in Dallas. Low-fat, high-carbohydrate diets, on the other hand, can lower HDL. But, on a low-fat, high-carbohydrate diet, your LDL will fall far faster, and your ratio of total cholesterol to HDL will actually improve.

The Greeks and Japanese were not only less likely candidates for heart disease, they also were (and are) less likely to get breast, colon, and prostate cancer. What's more, a recent study from Spain found that women who consumed the most olive oil were a third less likely to develop breast cancer than women who ate the least olive oil. It's not clear whether it's the olive oil or the fruits and vegetables in the Mediterranean diet that are protective. Either way, both the Mediterranean and low-fat diets seem to lower the risk of cancer.

Weight gain is the most controversial part of the Mediterranean diet. Keep in mind that while the Greeks consumed large amounts of olive oil, they also led very active lifestyles, burning 3,500 to 5,000 calories a day. It's amazing that most people assume olive oil in any amount has health benefits. At the end of a nutrition seminar for senior citizens several years ago, a woman came up to me and said, "My husband and I have been using olive oil for six months now to lower cholesterol. We put it in our juice each morning, I fry all our meats with it, and we use about a gallon a month. Isn't that great!" she exclaimed. This unfortunate woman had read in the paper that olive oil lowered cholesterol and assumed that the more she ate, the lower her cholesterol would go. The real reason she wanted to talk to me was that both she and her husband had gained about fifteen pounds each—and they didn't know why!

The Mediterranean diet is far more than using olive oil instead of salad dressing and margarine. You've got to substitute the oil for foods like meat, poultry, cheese, and pastries. That's the only way to keep your saturated fat as low as it was in the Mediterranean diet. It's a fairly simple eating style. The focus is on dry beans, vegetables, fruits, grains, olive oil, nuts, minimal amounts of meat, and wine in moderation. Each of these simple foods provides major nutritional benefits. Because beans are eaten daily, the Mediterranean diet is high in soluble fiber. It is unlikely that the Mediterranean diet would meet current dietary recommendations for calcium and possibly iron. And there's no avoiding the fact that these folks who lived a generation ago had very different exercise and activity patterns than today's Americans.

Traditional Chinese Medicine (TCM)

TCM is a comprehensive health system that includes diet, herbs, exercise, traditional Asian martial arts, and massage. The fundamental principle of health is the invisible energy force called qi (CHEE). These energy forces flow through your body along a series of channels called meridians. In addition to qi, your body consists of the material components of moisture and blood and the immaterial parts called spirit and essence. The balance of five elements—qi, moisture, blood, spirit, and essence—is essential for optimal health.

Traditional Chinese Medicine relies on herbs, acupuncture, nutrition, body work, and exercise to balance your body's energy. Further divisions are made for networks of organs: the kidneys, heart, lungs, liver, and spleen. These systems are responsible for regulating and distributing the five elements. A practitioner of TCM will spend considerable time examining your body for imbalances in these systems. A pulse check can last many minutes while you are checked for pulse quality, rhythm, and strength. Your tongue and ears will also be closely inspected for signs of disturbance. When these data are combined with information about your medical and family history and usual lifestyle, a personalized healing program will be developed for you.

Traditional Chinese Medicine Categories

Flavor of Food	Effects and Properties
Sour	acts on liver; astringent and stops abnormal discharges
Bitter	affects the heart; removes excess heat, eliminates dampness, removes toxic substances, corrects the direction of qi, purges pathogenic fire
Spicy	directed to the lungs; disperses and promotes qi circulation
Salty	acts on kidneys; reduces hard lumps or masses in the body
Sweet	works on spleen; nourishes, invigorates, regulates qi and blood, relieves spasms and pain
Bland	targets stomach and spleen; promotes urination, strengthens spleen, eliminates dampness

Season	Effects and Recommended Foods
Autumn	dry weather; eat yin foods to moisten the lungs such as honey, sesame, dairy, apples, bananas, grapes, water chestnuts, pears, oranges, tangerines, radishes, kelp, and lotus root
Winter	cold weather; eat warm/hot foods such as lamb, ginger, pepper, onion, Chinese green onion, garlic, and green leafy vegetables
Spring	liver is in hyperfunctioning state, digestion and spleen functions are suppressed. Choose sweet, hot, and sour flavors to nourish the spleen, such as Chinese dates, honey, malt sugar, and carrots
Summer	weaker digestion; eat light foods that are easily digested such as watermelon and a variety of vegetables

Acupuncture is perhaps the most controversial aspect of TCM. Acupuncture needles are quite different from the needles you've been stuck with for vaccines or injections. The tiny stainless steel needles are so thin, you might not even notice they've been placed in strategic areas to rechannel your circulation. Each of the five organ networks has a corresponding set of meridians. Depending on your specific health problem, the needles may be placed for just a few minutes or up to an hour.

Vegetarian Eating—Nuts about Veggies

If you think that vegetarians eat a lot of weird food, think again. Macaroni and cheese, peanut butter and jelly sandwiches, tomato soup, breakfast cereal, and eggs are all food options for some vegetarians.

Vegetarians are less likely to develop chronic degenerative conditions that plague the rest of the American population: diabetes, high blood pressure, heart disease, and obesity. But just leaving out animal foods does not undo all the "wrongs" of the typical American diet. Without sufficient knowledge of nutrient needs, going on a vegetarian diet because it seems politically correct or the right thing to do could lead to vitamin and mineral deficiencies.

Protein isn't a problem. Plant sources alone can provide plenty of protein. In fact, vegans (the strictest of all type of vegetarian eaters) tend not to be deficient in protein. A cup and a half of pasta alone contains 11 grams of protein. Add in 1 cup of broccoli and ½ cup of tomato sauce, and the protein tally jumps to 19 grams. For years, vegetarians were counseled to eat complementary proteins—two or more foods that contain different combinations of the complete proteins found in meat (whole-grain bread and peanut butter is one example). Today we know there's no need to eat complementary foods together, so long as you follow a varied diet each day.

One of the biggest pluses of eating a plant-based diet is that plant foods help keep fat content low. But you don't have to go completely vegetarian to enjoy the health benefits of a vegetarian lifestyle. Small changes in the proportions of foods from plants and animals will give the same results. Cut back on portion sizes of meat and fill the gap with extra vegetables, grains, or legumes.

Of the 6 to 8 million Americans who call themselves vegetarian, 90 percent eat eggs and cheese and drink milk. People who eat fish and white meats are not really vegetarians. Each type has a different name, depending on what foods they include: ovo (eats eggs), lacto (eats dairy products), lacto-ovo (eats eggs and dairy products). Vegans are vegetarians who do not use other animal products, and by-products such as eggs, dairy products, honey, leather, fur, silk, wool, cosmetics, and soaps derived from animal products, according to the Vegetarian Resource Group. People choose a vegan lifestyle for different reasons. Some have moral opposition to use of animal products; others feel it's better for our world environment not to rely on animal resources. Some believe a plant-based diet is more healthful than one that includes animal foods. Vegan diets require a real commitment of time: time to learn about food and nutrition, time to plan menus, and time to prepare foods.

Vegetarian Pyramid

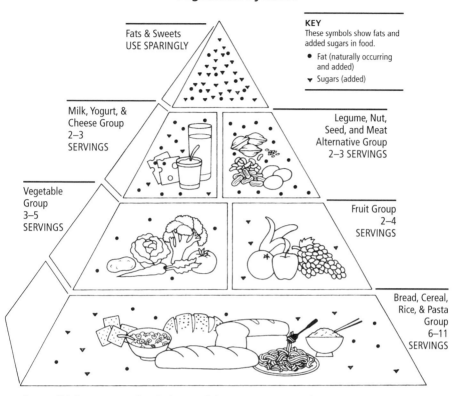

Fats & Sweets
USE SPARINGLY

KEY
These symbols show fats and added sugars in food.
- ● Fat (naturally occurring and added)
- ▾ Sugars (added)

Milk, Yogurt, & Cheese Group
2–3 SERVINGS

Legume, Nut, Seed, and Meat Alternative Group
2–3 SERVINGS

Vegetable Group
3–5 SERVINGS

Fruit Group
2–4 SERVINGS

Bread, Cereal, Rice, & Pasta Group
6–11 SERVINGS

Source: U.S. Department of Agriculture and the U.S. Department of Health and Human Services

Where Can You Get Vegetarian Foods?

Source	Percentage that Offer Complete Vegetarian Meals
Worksite Cafeterias	17%
Hospital Cafeterias	23%
Universities	27%
Restaurants	40%
Secondary Schools	80%
Contract Foodservice Management Companies	90%
Correctional Feeding (prisons)	100%

Source: *Food Industry Newsletter,* May 4, 1998

LINK UP to **http://www.vrg.org** for information on vegetarian nutrition and recipes from the Vegetarian Resource Group.

THE YOUNG AND THE MEATLESS

French fries and soft drinks aren't exactly what come to mind when you think vegetarian. But that's what some vegetarian teens—the fastest-growing segment of U.S. vegetarians—order when they eat out. Parents' concerns about the nutritional adequacy of a teen vegetarian diet are often justified, according to Cyndi Reeser, chair of the vegetarian nutrition practice group of the American Dietetic Association. "Teens who adopt a vegetarian eating pattern do so with strong convictions and few nutrient resources," says Reeser. Low intakes of iron and calcium are common in all teenage girls. Zinc and vitman B_{12} may be of special concern for vegetarian teens who are vegans. Reeser recommends parents offer support by stocking foods with teen appeal: cereal with milk or soy milk, bagels, hummus and pita bread, bean dip and tortillas, low-fat tortilla chips and salsa, ready-to-eat lentil and pea soups, veggie burgers, yogurt, and dried fruit and nut mixes. A daily multivitamin and mineral supplement may also be a good option.

Offer to give your teen a nutrition consultation with a registered dietitian and ask if you can sit in on the session, suggests Reeser. Vegetarian teens most at risk are those who eat a limited variety of foods, skip meals frequently, avoid entire categories of foods, or are preoccupied with thinness and body image.

Nutrient-Based Eating Styles

40-30-30, 55-15-30, and 65-15-15. No, these are not good picks for the lottery, they are number sequences that represent some popular combinations of the proportion of carbohydrate to protein to fat in an "ideal" diet. There is no perfect, one-size-fits-all recommendation for how to choose food by the numbers.

High Protein Usually Means High Fat

Men love high-protein diets. These eating plans grant permission to chow down on beefy steaks and drink beer. Minnesota Vikings football coach Dennis Green's high-protein diet gained such local acclaim that Minnesota grocery stores started stocking pork rinds. Customers were demanding the never-before-stocked snack item because "Denny eats it." Pork rinds were big on Green's "high-protein diet," and he loved sharing how much he enjoyed eating these grease-laden globs of pig skin.

The American College of Sports Medicine, the American Dietetic Association, the Women's Sports Foundation, and the Cooper Institute for Aerobics Research have released a joint statement saying that high-protein plans are the answer neither for weight loss nor for athletic performance and can cause harm. Here are their reasons:

- Protein should only make up 10 to 15 percent of calories per day.
- High-protein plans usually recommend 40 percent of calories from carbohydrates, 30 percent from protein, and 30 percent from fat; this provides a diet inadequate in some major nutrients, particularly carbohydrates.
- Although some people manage to lose weight on a high-protein plan, it is only because they eat so few calories.

The health and diet aisle of your local bookstore is chock full of titles such as *Protein Power, The Zone, Healthy for Life, The 5 Day Miracle Diet,* and *Dr. Atkins' New Diet Revolution,* all featuring protein-powered diets. Such diets have a decidedly familiar ring. They are making a comeback from their heyday in the 1970s. But these "new" high-protein diets are the same old bad news. Following such an eating plan can result in an immediate and dramatic loss of body fluid. It's rewarding to see the pounds drops quickly at first, and most dieters think they've lost a lot of body fat, not just water. The build up of ketones caused by high-protein diets can cause fatigue, weakness, headache, irritability, bad breath, dehydration, and kidney trouble. Ketogenic diets are especially dangerous for older people or those with untreated diabetes. Here's a quick rundown on the current best-selling high-protein fad diets:

- *Dr. Atkins' New Diet Revolution:* The original high-protein diet guru continues to rehash his high-protein, relatively high-fat diet with carbohydrate levels ranging from a meager 15 gm (1 serving of fruit, bread, rice, or pasta) to a barely adequate 60 gm a day for beginning dieters.
- *The 5 Day Miracle Diet,* by Adelle Puhn, is a bit more generous with carbohydrates, but not much. Women are advised to eat starchy vegetables, potatoes, or beans only on alternate days—either for lunch or dinner, but not both. What about pasta? Not more than twice a week and only at dinner.
- The diet in Barry Sears's *The Zone* is referred to as "40-30-30" by those in the know, where the 40 represents a goal of 40 percent of total calories from protein, plus 30 percent from carbohydrates, and 30 percent from fat. This is still considerably more protein (two to three times) and less carbohydrate than most nutritionists recommend. However, you're unlikely to experience a buildup of ketones on this diet.

So what's the alternative? It may not be a hot new trend, but eating plenty of fruits, vegetables, and whole grains along with moderate amounts of lean meats and low-fat dairy foods, coupled with regular physical activity, is the safest bet for keeping off unwanted pounds.

Moderate Low-Fat Eating

Americans are eating fewer calories from fat, but that may not be all good news. Many people are just replacing high-fat diets with diets heavy in processed carbohydrates—low-fat chips, cookies, and other snack foods. What you need to do is eat more fruits and vegetables containing beneficial nutrients. Today's focus on the 30 percent of calories from fat has failed to help most people make better food choices. Fat is just one factor to review on a food label. If a food is fat-free but also devoid of any other nutrients, it offers no positive benefit. The proliferation of fat-free and low-fat products has offered more opportunity to eat poorly.

High-Carbohydrate, Very Low-Fat Diets

With 15 percent of calories from fat, these diets are very difficult to follow because variety and amounts of many foods and food groups are severely restricted. The Pritikin diet is perhaps the best example of severe fat restriction. There is no dispute that for some, this combination of foods can actually stop or reverse symptoms of heart disease. This eating style is great for these folks, but not to be recommended as an overall healthful diet. Why? Studies in progress are helping to explain why not everyone reduces their risk for heart disease by going on low-fat diets. The answers aren't all in yet. According to nutrition and obesity expert C. Wayne Calloway, M.D., one-fourth of the U.S. population develops insulin resistance on these high-carbohydrate diets—a condition that frequently leads to diabetes. "The trend for the future is more targeted dietary prescriptions for individuals, not one-size-fits-all diets," says Calloway.

Choose Your Own Style

Considering all the data you collected in Chapter 1 and what you understand so far, it's time to plan your own eating style. To implement any broad guidelines may seem overwhelming. You need to make healthful choices that fit your lifestyle so you can do the things you want to do. The "It's All About You" campaign offers some simple, action-oriented tips to provide easy and manageable ways to help change your behavior and integrate basic dietary guidelines into your life.

It's All About You

Be Realistic—Make small changes over time in what you eat and the level of activity you do. After all, small steps work better than giant leaps.

- Park your car in the farthest spot. You'll walk more and burn extra calories.
- For lower-fat chili or tacos, put cooked ground beef in a strainer and rinse briefly with hot water. Drain well and continue with your recipe.

- To cut calories and fat, use a cooking spray instead of oil to sauté foods.
- Check the vending machine for lower-fat goodies like pretzels, bagels, low-fat yogurt, fresh fruit, and skim milk.
- Shopping on the run? Choose products that say "low," "high," or "reduced" on the label—these terms are easy to see and mean what they say.

Be Adventurous—Expand your tastes to enjoy a variety of foods.
- Try a fruit or vegetable you haven't had before. Make it a monthly goal.
- Enjoy a meal at a Thai, Indian, or Japanese restaurant.
- Prepare one new recipe each month from a favorite magazine or newspaper article.
- Dig into a different grain: couscous, bulgur, or quinoa, for instance.
- Pick up a food you don't normally buy each time you shop.
- Try imaginative low-fat snacks such as fruit kabobs or air-popped popcorn seasoned lightly with herbs or grated cheese.
- Strive to eat the number of servings recommended from each of the food groups in the Food Guide Pyramid.
- Choose an entree that is grilled or broiled when eating out.

Be Flexible—Go ahead and balance what you eat and the physical activity you do over several days. No need to worry about just one meal or one day.
- Eat a lighter breakfast and lunch to plan for "pizza with the works" for dinner.
- Don't pack on extra pounds during vacations. Work in plenty of walking, biking, hiking, or active games to balance out special vacation meals.
- Did you splurge on a "soup to nuts" special occasion meal? No problem. Eat lighter and move more for a few days afterward.
- No need to track every food you eat. But for foods you eat often, check the percent DV (daily value) column on food labels and balance high-fat choices with lower-fat ones.
- Enjoy a walk with a friend or family member before dinner.

Be Sensible—Enjoy all foods, just don't overdo it.
- Slow down! It takes twenty minutes for your brain to send the signal that you've had enough to eat.
- When served oversize portions in restaurants, eat half and take the rest home to enjoy the next day.
- Have only one helping and enjoy every bite.

- Make your ice-cream cone a single, not a double, dip.
- Serve your snacks on a plate to control the amount you eat rather than eating straight out of the bag.

Be Active—Walk the dog, don't just watch the dog walk.

- Set your goal at thirty minutes of moderate activity most days. In ten-minute increments, it's easier.
- Take a brisk ten-minute walk on your lunch break. You'll feel good and have more energy, too.
- Hop off the bus a few blocks early and walk briskly the rest of the way.
- Keep active around the house: sweep the garage, scrub the floors, vacuum the rugs, or trim the shrubs. It all helps you get fit—and the house will look great, too.
- Try a fun new activity. How about ballroom dancing, Roller-Blading, ice skating, or line dancing?
- Get energized. Take a brisk ten-minute walk in the morning, at lunch, and after dinner to total thirty minutes a day.
- Climb the stairs instead of riding the elevator. You'll be more fit without adding additional time to your fitness routine.

5

Vitamins

"If you eat a balanced diet, you don't need supplements." This has been the advice of most health professionals for decades. It's time for a change. Substantial evidence shows that intakes greater than the Recommended Dietary Allowances (RDAs) of specific vitamins and minerals reduce the risk of particular diseases. The evaluation of your diet from Chapter 1 will help you determine which supplements are needed for optimal health. An appropriate intake of the right vitamins and minerals will help you feel and look your best no matter what your age. You may be able to significantly reduce the risk of chronic, crippling diseases that steal your energy, enjoyment, and enthusiasm for life. Supplements are not magic bullets, nor will they neutralize the impact of a high-fat, low-fiber diet of overly processed foods. Don't rely on supplements as a nutritional shortcut—you won't come out a winner.

Recent scientific studies have begun to focus on intake levels above the amount needed to prevent nutritional deficiencies in an effort to optimize health. Example include studies which report that particular nutrients have antioxidant effects that protect against heart disease, certain cancers, and cataracts. They're called antioxidants because they prevent damage from a process known as oxidation. If not controlled, oxidation results in damage to cells. Niacin used alone and in combination with other medications lowers blood cholesterol. Calcium in amounts higher than traditionally recommended can slow the development of osteoporosis and may lower blood pressure in some people.

Despite these dramatic findings, there's little official acknowledgment that supplements have value except for use by a small number of groups including:

- newborns routinely given a single dose of vitamin K to prevent abnormal bleeding.
- pregnant and breast-feeding women's increased needs for most nutrients.

- women of childbearing age who benefit from folate supplements.
- women with heavy menstrual periods who may need iron supplementation.
- those on very low-calorie diets who simply don't eat enough to get essential nutrients.
- vegans (vegetarians who eat no animal products) who often don't eat enough foods rich in calcium, iron, zinc, and vitamin B$_{12}$.
- people with chronic illnesses that affect how they absorb nutrients.

Supplement use by anyone else is often regarded as unscientific and at best a waste of money. Eating nutrient-rich foods is clearly the preferred way to consume vitamins and minerals. But anyone eating less than 1,500 calories a day simply can't eat enough food to meet even the minimum standards for some nutrients. And to be realistic, you may not eat the right combination of foods to meet minimum intake standards and may not be close to preventive amounts.

Deplorable Diets

The U.S. Committee on Dietary Allowances estimates that many Americans consume 30 percent or more of their calories from foods that provide few, if any, vitamins or minerals. A 1998 study of the dietary sources of nutrients in U.S. adults reports similar results:

Food Category	Percent of Total Calories
Cakes, cookies, quick breads, and doughnuts	5.5
Soft drinks/sodas	4.1
Salad dressings/mayonnaise	3.1
Margarine	3.0
Sugars/syrups/jams	2.8
Alcoholic beverages	2.5
Potato chips/corn chips/popcorn	2.1
Oils	1.0
Fruit drinks (not juice)	1.0

Source: *Journal of the American Dietetic Association,* 1998

VITAMIN-MINERAL REVELATIONS

Vitamin and mineral knowledge is in its infancy. Less than one hundred years ago the first vitamin, vitamin A, was discovered. Initially, research focused on finding the smallest amount of a nutrient that would prevent common deficiency diseases like scurvy (vitamin C deficiency) and beriberi (thiamin deficiency). Then, as more nutrients were identified, how they interacted became important. Today we're on the threshold of a whole new era identifying more unique categories of nutrients and learning how they optimize health and thwart disease.

Animal, Vegetable, or Mineral?

Vitamins are chemical compounds containing carbon, which is necessary for growth, health, metabolism, and physical well-being. Vitamins are found in plant and animal foods. Some vitamins are essential parts of enzymes—the molecules that help complete chemical reactions. Other vitamins form parts of hormones—substances that promote and protect overall health and reproduction.

Plants make almost all of their own vitamins. Animals can create their own vitamins, too. For example, cats and dogs manufacture vitamin C. Humans must obtain vitamins from foods, produce them in their skin or liver, or make them with intestinal bacteria. For example, vitamin D can be synthesized by skin when exposed to sunlight; vitamin K and biotin are made from bacteria in the colon; and niacin is converted from the amino acid tryptophan in your gut.

There are facts we know about vitamins and minerals:

- Vitamins and minerals don't provide calories or energy.
- All necessary vitamins and minerals can be found in food.
- All vitamins are organic since they contain the element carbon.
- All minerals are inorganic since they do not contain carbon.
- If you don't consume a particular vitamin or mineral, a deficiency will result over time.
- For most vitamins and minerals, the best form or most available source is the food we eat.

From A to Zinc

It's not surprising if vitamins and minerals seem a little foreign. Unlike most common things we measure, nutrients are tallied using the metric system of grams, milligrams, and micrograms. These are very tiny measurements—one gram is about the weight of a small paper clip. In fact, your total vitamin and mineral needs for a day would barely add up to ⅛ teaspoon. To make it even more complex, some nutrients are measured in more than one way. For example, vitamin A is counted in retinol equivalents (REs), international units (IUs), and beta-carotene equivalencies. In this book the most common unit of measure is used whenever possible, so that it's easier for you to compare food and supplement labels.

GO FIGURE: NUTRIENT MEASURES AND CONVERSIONS

5 grams = 1 teaspoon

14 grams = ½ ounce = 1 tablespoon = 3 teaspoons

28 grams = 1 ounce = 2 tablespoons

10,000 micrograms = 1,000 milligrams = 1 gram

1 IU of vitamin A = .3 mcg retinol = .6 mcg beta-carotene

1 mg alpha-tocopherol acetate = 1 IU

Alphabet Soup of Standards

To confuse matters more, there are a variety of scientific standards, none of them adequate, to help sort out how much of a particular nutrient is desirable. Sometimes government and other standards complement each other; occasionally they conflict. Policymakers and health organizations need to carefully review and update their recommendations on supplement use to provide consumers with credible and consistent information. This takes time, so sometimes information gets out in the media long before enough science is available to make a clear recommendation. We've included all of the government's recommended nutrient charts in one of the appendices of this book.

Recommended Dietary Allowances (RDAs) were once the gold standard of nutrient recommendations. The RDAs tell us how much of each nutrient the population as a whole needs to prevent deficiency states. But even its creators admit that the numbers are not as meaningful as you might hope. The RDAs were designed by the National Academy of Sciences in 1941 for the War Department. They were used as a guide to feeding U.S. soldiers, and the basic concepts haven't changed much in the last fifty years. If you ate close to 100 percent of the RDAs for the nutrients listed, chances were good you had a balanced diet; that is, if you were a healthy person to start with. If you consume the RDA for vitamin C (60 mg), for instance, you will have a very low risk of scurvy.

Adequate Intakes (AIs) are the "best guesses" of experts when not enough science is available to make a formal RDA. Based on a combination of research and observation, they offer a range of intakes that should keep most people healthy.

Daily Values (DVs and %DVs) were invented when the food label was redesigned in 1992. Many people are understandably confused by these new standards. If you are healthy and fit and eat exactly 2,000 calories a day, then the DVs are tailored with you in mind. Since most of us don't eat exactly a 2,000-calorie diet, you may need more or less than 100 percent of the DVs.

Dietary Reference Intakes (DRIs) are the new kids on the block and are being promoted as a major leap forward in nutrition science. It's no longer feasible to have a single reference number for each nutrient. DRIs take a broader perspective, examining each nutrient's role in decreasing your risk of developing chronic diseases. They also set an upper level of intake to protect you from the risk of toxicity. The new goal is more than protection against deficiency; it aims at lowering of your risk of major chronic diseases. Currently DRIs are available for B vitamins and vitamins and minerals involved in bone health such as calcium and magnesium. It is expected that in the near future, DRIs will be developed for all nutrients.

Tolerable Upper Intake Levels (ULs) are the maximum amount of a nutrient that won't hurt you, if you are a healthy person to begin with. ULs are not intended to be a recommended level of intake but a marker for reasonable safety for those who want to "push the envelope." For most nutrients, this number refers to total intake from food, fortified food, and nutritional supplements.

More Is Not Always Better

A megadose of a nutrient is typically any amount greater than ten times your RDA. At this level nutrients act differently in your body. Megadoses of some nutrients have significant druglike effects. The most frequent side effects from taking too many supplemental nutrients are vague. They include common symptoms such as headache, weakness, fatigue, nausea, and vomiting. Often these are the same early symptoms of many other illnesses, including vitamin deficiency. If you notice any early warning signs, be sure to tell your health care provider you are taking supplements. It's a good idea to compile a list of all the supplements you're taking and share this with your doctor at every visit.

Fortified foods have nutrients added to them during processing. Federal law requires manufacturers to add specific nutrients to certain foods. For example, milk processors add vitamins A and D. Food companies can choose to selectively add almost any nutrient to increase the appeal of a food. For instance, orange juice and rice both come in calcium-fortified versions. Getting nutrients from fortified foods is similar to taking a supplement. There is no guarantee that the form of the nutrient added contains all the known and unknown benefits of eating a real food source.

Nutrients in a Nutshell

With so many gaps in knowledge and differences between individual needs, it's difficult to weed through the tangle of data that continues to grow around vitamins and minerals. The following vitamin profiles offer a framework for determining if you would benefit from an increased intake. Chapter 6 does the same for minerals.

This section will dispel myths and accurately summarize the facts and current findings on each vitamin, detailing several important aspects such as:

- Up-to-date information. A quick review of interesting facts, current knowledge, and research trends.
- A brief description of each nutrient and why you need it.
- Recommendations for optimal intake. These levels may be higher than the current RDA or DV, based on the analysis of scientific studies, review papers, and interviews with leading experts. The unit of measure (IU, mg, mcg, etc.) listed is the most common way each vitamin is sold.
- Natural food sources. These are foods that provide at least 25 percent of the RDA in just one serving. If you are low in any particular nutrient, scan this list for quick, concentrated food ideas.
- Fortified foods. You should eat foods that are naturally high in nutrients. If you can't or won't, try foods that have those particular nutrients added during processing. Eating a fortified food is a second-rate choice; taking a supplement is third on the list.
- Minimum toxic doses. This is the smallest amount of a nutrient that can cause side effects ranging from annoying to life-threatening.
- Selected studies. These are quick glimpses of highlights from current research related to a particular nutrient, not a comprehensive list of studies. Journal or report citations are provided if you want to look them up yourself. When you look up one of these studies, check the reference list the authors provide if you want to do more digging.

Vitamins don't have glamorous or exciting names. The first one was named fat-soluble A and the second, water-soluble B. When riboflavin was discovered in 1926, it was found dissolvable in water and was called water-soluble B_2. So the original B vitamin became B_1. Things really got jumbled when someone figured out that B_1 was two vitamins— thiamin and niacin. Thiamin kept the B_1 name, and since B_2 was already taken, niacin was dubbed B_3. And so the story goes. Why isn't there vitamin B_4 or B_9? Overzealous researchers sometimes named a compound a vitamin and then later realized their mistake. It was too messy to continually reassign numbers. Eventually vitamin researchers wisened up and started giving names instead of numbers to their discoveries.

FAT-SOLUBLE NUTRIENTS

Fat-soluble vitamins include vitamins A, D, E, and K. They are unique because they are found and stored in fatty tissue. You must eat some fat so these nutrients can be absorbed from foods. Because these vitamins are

TOXIC TALK

Both one-time overdoses or prolonged overconsumption can cause health impairments. Toxic doses of vitamins and minerals rarely result from eating too much food; oversupplementation is the culprit. There are three types of vitamin/mineral toxicity:

- Acute or sudden toxicity occurs from one very big dose or from several huge doses over a few days. You get sick right away.
- Chronic toxicity develops after weeks or months of habitually taking extreme levels of a nutrient. For example, megadoses (amounts ten times or more the RDA) of vitamin B_6 can cause nerve disorders and skin rashes. Permanent damage may occur with some forms of chronic toxicity. Most people who develop toxic reactions to supplements don't have a clue it's their vitamin or mineral intake that's causing the problem. What commonly happens is you go through an expensive and exhaustive series of tests. Finally, you remember to tell your doctor that you take supplements. If you're lucky, your symptoms go away shortly after you stop them.
- Teratogenic toxicity refers to harmful changes in a baby's development that occur during pregnancy. Pregnant women risk miscarriage or severe birth defects if they take large amounts of certain supplements, such as vitamin A.

held in fatty tissue, you don't need to replenish them every day—you can "save them up" over time. However, fat-soluble vitamins have a much greater potential for being toxic, since storage in body fat is almost unlimited. It's almost impossible to overdose on fat-soluble vitamins from food sources—unless you have a hankering for polar bear liver! Arctic explorers sought out polar bear and seal liver to help extend their marginal food rations. Unfortunately, arctic animals like polar bears and seals store vitamin A in amounts that are toxic and often fatal to humans.

Vitamin A

Vitamins are not the simple structures scientists once thought they were. Continuing research shows that many nutrients, like vitamin A, are a family of compounds. The three main types of vitamin A are carotenoids, retinol, and retinal. The carotenoids (ka-ROT-en-oids) are a group of more than 500 individual carotenes, the most popular member being beta-carotene. You can see them in the natural coloring of foods: the red in a pepper, the orange in a carrot, and the yellow in squash. Some vitamin A is masked so it can be found in a few leafy green vegetables as well. The only adverse effect of eating too many carotenoids over time is that your skin may take on a light orange glow. That's because the fat in skin cells store excesses of vitamin A. If you cut back on your intake, the unusual color will disappear within two to six weeks.

Retinol and retinal are found in animal foods. They are ready to be used by the body as is. That's why they are sometimes referred to as pre-formed vitamin A. Your overall intake is the sum total of all types of vitamin A you consume.

Until recently only preformed vitamin A was typically found in supplement tablets. Now we know that beta-carotene and other carotenoids such as lycopene (LYE-co-peen) and lutein (LEW-tea-in) do more than just change into vitamin A. They also act as antioxidants. Lutein (from dark green leafy vegetables) has been shown to reduce the risk of cataracts. Tomatoes, watermelon, and grapefruit contain lycopene, which may protect men from prostate cancer.

Xerophthalmia (zeer-OH-thal-ME-ah) is the deficiency disease that results from too little vitamin A. When the mucous (moisture) membranes in the eye dry out, small particles of dirt settle there. Bacteria can enter the vulnerable eye through the scratches caused by these dirt particles. White blood cells, which help fight infection, start attacking bacteria in the scratches and cause lesions. As the lesions grow, blindness can result. Other signs of vitamin A deficiency include respiratory infection, stunted growth, and extremely dry skin (keratinization).

Recent research suggests that optimal intakes of vitamin A may strengthen the immune system and fend off certain cancers. Vitamin A helps protect body surfaces designed to keep infection and disease out. These special surfaces include your skin and the moist lining of your mouth, throat, and digestive tract. Vitamin A's influence on immunity may be one of the ways it helps prevent the initiation or growth of cancer cells.

Why you need it: vitamin A is critical for normal growth and healthy development. It's especially key in stimulating night and color vision. That's because vitamin A helps maintain the protective layers of the skin, including the eyes. Vitamin A combines with a special protein in your eye that improves night vision.

For optimal health: 5,000 IU/day of vitamin A

Best natural food sources: carrot, cantaloupe, kale, mango, peppers, squash, sweet potato, and turnip greens

Fortified foods: low-fat and skim milk, margarine, and ready-to-eat cereals

Minimum toxic dose: 6,500 IU or 15 to 30 mg or more/day of vitamin A may cause blurred vision, diarrhea, headaches, irritability, muscle weakness, skin scaling or peeling, and vomiting. In growing children excess vitamin A can cause premature bone closures that result in deformities. Too much vitamin A is also known to cause stunted growth in children. During pregnancy vitamin A toxicity causes a variety of birth defects.

Selected Studies

- People who eat at restaurants at least once a week consume fewer carotenoids than people who eat at home (*American Journal of Public Health,* February 1997). That's because most restaurant meals lack deep yellow and orange vegetables rich in vitamin A. If you eat out frequently, be sure to eat lots of vitamin A–rich foods at home and for snacks.

- Almost 23,000 pregnant women consuming various levels of vitamin A were contacted after the birth of their children. Women who had combined food and supplement intakes of 15,000 IUs of preformed vitamin A had a 3.5 times increased risk for birth defects compared to women who typically consumed just 5,000 IU. Those women who took 10,000 IU or more of vitamin A from supplements alone had a 4.8 times higher rate of infants born with a birth defect (*New England Journal of Medicine,* November 1995). If you might get pregnant, don't take extra amounts of vitamin A from supplements beyond what's in a daily multivitamin tablet.

- An increased intake of beta-carotene by healthy, breast-feeding women increases the supply of beta-carotene available to their infants (*American Journal of Clinical Nutrition,* February 1998). This is one more study that proves breast milk is the best milk for babies.

Vitamin D

A stroll in the park, tending your garden, or watching the kids splash in the pool are some of the more pleasant ways to obtain vitamin D. Since you make your own vitamin D when you're in the sun, it's sometimes called the sunshine vitamin.

Vitamin D comes in three forms: calciferol (cal-SIFF-er-all), cholecalciferol (KO-lee-cal-SIFF-er-all), and ergocalciferol (UR-go-cal-SIFF-er-all). All can be made by exposing your skin to a sufficient amount of sunlight or artificial ultraviolet radiation. Vitamin D is also found in fortified milk and other dairy products. Vitamin D helps calcium be absorbed into the body. Without enough vitamin D, your body adapts by absorbing only 10 to 15 percent of all the calcium you take in. Too little vitamin D can speed up the development of the crippling bone disease osteoporosis. Occasionally, a vitamin D deficiency may cause slow, progressive hearing loss. If the bones in the inner ear become too weak or porous, they will not properly transmit sound waves. Sometimes this special type of hearing loss can be improved with an adequate intake of vitamin D.

Concern over sun-damaged skin and skin cancer has resulted in the increased use of sunscreens and sun-avoidance. If you shy away from the sun, you may not get enough vitamin D. There are many factors to consider when evaluating how reasonable it is to bask in the warmth of the sun in order to make your own vitamin D:

- Where you live. Check your latitude on the map on the next page. If you live in the southernmost half of the United States, chances are good that with regular outdoor time you can make and store plenty of vitamin D. If you live in the north, you should rely more on food sources of vitamin D.

- Season. In many northern climates it is impossible to have sufficient sun exposure in late fall, winter, and early spring due to the earth's distance from the sun.

- Sun protection. Sunscreens, clothing, hats, and other protective items block exposure to sunlight necessary to make vitamin D. Your skin must be exposed (the more the better) and free of any protective sunscreen for the sun to perform its magic. If you regularly apply sunscreen with a sun protection factor (SPF) of 8 or more, you won't make enough vitamin D from sun exposure.

- Mobility. If you stay indoors frequently or have extensive restrictions on activity (such as those in nursing homes or confined to bed), you probably aren't outdoors enough to soak up needed rays.

- Skin tone. Individuals with dark skin pigmentation have a higher melanin content and require a much longer exposure time (thirty to forty minutes, three to four times a week) than people with light skin tones (fifteen to twenty minutes, three to four times a week).

- Age. If you're over 70, your ability to make vitamin D from sun exposure is reduced by half. For instance, a fair-skinned child who plays outdoors year-round would probably not need a supplement of vitamin D, whereas a homebound elderly woman would require fortified foods or pills to prevent potential weakening of bone tissue.

Vitamin D isn't just for bones anymore. As important as bone health is, vitamin D's role in regulating how much calcium stays in your blood is just as critical. Calcium is important for the transmission of nerve impulses and is required for muscle contraction. Perhaps the most important muscle that needs calcium to work effectively is your heart.

If you regularly rely on laxatives (all types) or antacids with aluminum or magnesium (these lower calcium absorption), be aware because these products can lower the amount of vitamin D you absorb from foods. The cholesterol-lowering drug cholestyramine (Questran) also disrupts absorption and metabolism of vitamin D. Fat substitutes like Olean and the fat-blocking drug Xenical also limit the amount of fat-soluble nutrients your body is able to absorb. If you regularly consume any of these, you should take a multivitamin supplement.

Exposing Yourself to Vitamin D

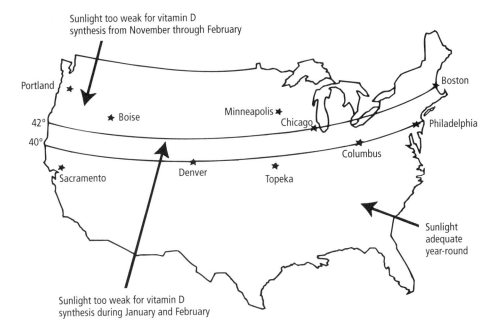

Exposure to sun must be without sunscreen in order
to manufacture your own vitamin D.

Why you need it: vitamin D is essential for helping calcium get into your bones. Without proper levels of vitamin D, you can't absorb enough calcium no matter how much you take in. This nutrient also helps maintain proper heart function.

For optimal health: 400 to 600 IU or 10 to 15 mcg/day of vitamin D. Diabetics and people who are exposed to high levels of toxic chemicals at work or air pollution where they live may need the higher optimal amounts.

Best natural food sources: tuna, salmon, and sardines

Fortified foods: milk, margarine, and butter

Minimum toxic dose: 1,000 IU or 25 mcg/day of vitamin D or more may cause constipation; headaches; nausea; high blood pressure; seizures; growth retardation; calcium deposits in the heart, blood vessels, and kidneys.

Selected Studies

- An eight-year study of 556 older men and women with osteoporosis found that those with low to moderate intakes (averaging 200 IU) and blood levels of vitamin D were three times more likely to have their symptoms worsen over time compared to those who had intakes of closer to 400 IU of vitamin D daily (*Annals of Internal Medicine,* September 1996). People with osteoporosis should carefully monitor the amount of vitamin D they consume to prevent pain and fractures.
- Another study showed what effects skin thickness, age, body fat, and sunlight can have on your blood levels of vitamin D (*American Journal of Clinical Nutrition,* 1993). The more risk factors you have, the harder it is for you to make or absorb vitamin D.

Vitamin E

If all the hype about vitamin E were true, you could live well past 100 and have the sex drive and youthful appearance of a teenager. Vitamin E is no fountain of youth, but it does provide significant health benefits. Working as an antioxidant, vitamin E protects various tissues from destruction by free radicals. Optimal intakes of vitamin E have also been linked to reduction of heart disease and cancer.

Unfortunately, vitamin E is one nutrient that is difficult to obtain in optimal amounts from moderate-calorie foods. It takes almost a pound of vegetables such as spinach, sweet potatoes, or peas to provide just 20 to 30 IU of vitamin E. Oils, nuts, and seeds are more concentrated sources of vitamin E, but they also contribute hefty amounts of fat grams and calories. Antacids decrease vitamin E absorption. If you habitually take antacids, you will need supplemental vitamin E.

NUTRITION ACTION Vitamin E is the only nutrient where the "natural" form is preferable over synthetic versions. Ignore the product label and read the ingredient list. Look for d-alpha-tocopherol. If you see dl-alpha-tocopherol, it's the synthetic version. The extra "l" makes all the difference. An easy way to remember what to avoid is dl = don't like.

Why you need it: vitamin E protects vitamin A and essential fatty acids from oxidation; prevents breakdown of body tissues. Vitamin E may also decrease heart attack risk and improve immunity.

For optimal health: 50 to 400 IU/day of vitamin E from foods or the natural form of the vitamin

Best natural food sources: almonds, hazelnuts (filberts), peanut butter, rice bran oil, shrimp, sunflower seeds, wheat germ, and wheat germ oil

Fortified foods: ready-to-eat cereals

Minimum toxic dose: 800 to 1,000 IU/day of vitamin E or more may cause breast tenderness, depression, diarrhea, double vision, fatigue, intestinal cramping, mood swings, and weak muscles. High doses can also interfere with the effectiveness of anticoagulant (blood-thinning) medicines that are prescribed to prevent blood clotting. Continued high intakes deplete vitamin A stores.

Selected Studies

- A study of 87,000 nurses found that women who took vitamin E supplements of 100 IU a day for at least two years had a 31 percent reduced risk of nonfatal heart attacks and deaths from coronary heart disease (*New England Journal of Medicine,* May 1993). Women at risk for heart disease should consider supplemental vitamin E.

- A study of 39,000 male health professionals found that men who took vitamin E supplements of at least 100 IU a day had a reduced risk of nonfatal heart attacks and deaths from coronary heart disease (*New England Journal of Medicine,* May 1993). Men with a family history of heart disease should consider supplemental vitamin E.

- A study of 2,002 people at Cambridge University found that men with existing heart disease who took a supplement of 400 to 800 IU of vitamin E daily for a year and a half reduced their risk of nonfatal heart attacks by 77 percent (*Lancet,* June 1997). The levels of vitamin E in this study are much higher than others. Try to eat foods rich in vitamin E instead of relying only on supplements.

- Data from a 1986 study of 34,000 postmenopausal women from Iowa examined at the University of Minnesota found that women who ate diets high in vitamin E had a 62 percent reduction of risk for heart disease. Vitamin E supplements didn't seem to lower the risk, possibly because few women in this study took them (*New England Journal of Medicine,* May 1996). It's tough to get optimal amounts of vitamin E just from foods. This study helps support the food-first principle. Women who had "pretty good" vitamin E intakes from foods fared better than those who did not.

Vitamin K

You don't hear much about vitamin K, but it is important. Most notably it helps your blood to clot and helps form bone tissue. Extra amounts of vitamin K are frequently needed by those on long-term antibiotic therapy and anyone who does not metabolize fat normally.

If you've ever had a baby, you might remember that almost all newborns are given an injection of vitamin K shortly before they leave the hospital. That's because newborns have not yet developed normal, healthy bacteria in their digestive tract that help produce one of the three forms of vitamin K called K2 (menaquione).

There are two other types of this nutrient. Vitamin K1 (phylloquinone) is found in foods and is also made by bacteria in your gut. K_3 (menadione) is a synthetic form of vitamin K found in the liver and is the most active form of the three. Most Americans consume more than the RDA of vitamin K. That makes deficiency quite rare. Some calcium supplements also contain vitamin K.

Why you need it: vitamin K controls blood clotting, maintains bone, and helps heal bone fractures.

For optimal health: 65 to 200 mcg/day of vitamin K

Best natural food sources: asparagus, broccoli, brussels sprouts, cabbage, collard greens, endive, green apples, kale, red leaf lettuce, Swiss chard, and watercress

Fortified foods: no food is fortified at 25 percent of the RDA

Minimum toxic dose: not known. May cause impaired liver function in those with advanced liver disease; jaundice and brain damage in infants. Large intakes of vitamin K can interact with the prescription drug wafarin (Coumadin).

Selected Studies

- Women who consume low levels of vitamin K have a greater risk of hip fractures than women who consume high or moderate levels of this nutrient (*American Journal of Clinical Nutrition,* January 1999). A single large salad of dark green leafy vegetables can provide all the extra vitamin K you need.

- A meta-analysis of six controlled clinical trials was evaluated to determine the safest and most effective method of administering vitamin K to infants to prevent hemorrhagic disease. No link with childhood cancer, as had been suggested by other research, was found (*Canadian Medical Association Journal,* February 1996). There is no compelling reason to change the current practice of administering vitamin K to newborns.

WATER-SOLUBLE VITAMINS

The eight B vitamins plus vitamin C make up the water-soluble nutrients. Unlike fat-soluble nutrients, these can't go into long-term storage. B and C vitamins get used up or washed out of the body quickly via urine and sweat. Because they are so fragile, it's easy to lose water-soluble nutrients before you even open your mouth to put them in. That's because exposure to light, air, or heat during storage, processing, or cooking diminishes availability. It's important to carefully handle and prepare foods that contain B and C vitamins so you don't end up washing these nutrients down the drain or pouring them out with the cooking water.

Thiamin—Vitamin B$_1$

Unless you eat lots of raw fish or rely on overly processed foods, chances are you're getting plenty of thiamin (THYE-ah-min). However, if you regularly sashay up to the sushi bar, beware that lurking in your uncooked fish is thiaminase, an enzyme that inactivates the nutrient thiamin. Cooking will deactivate this pesky thiamin destroyer.

The thiamin deficiency disease beriberi (Sri Lankan for "I can't, I can't") is most commonly seen where white rice is a staple food. Symptoms of depression and weakness show up as quickly as ten days without thiamin in the diet. Other symptoms include weight loss, loss of appetite, irritability, tingling skin, and deep muscle pain.

U.S. grain products are enriched with thiamin. Don't wash or rinse pasta or rice before cooking or you'll cause thiamin to leach out into the water. If you happen to buy imported rice, it's usually not enriched and should be washed to sift out impurities. If you buy imported, unenriched white rice, be sure to eat plenty of other enriched grains.

Alcoholics have an increased risk for thiamin deficiency, since alcohol significantly diminishes the ability to absorb and use thiamin. Alcohol-related thiamin deficiency leads to a cluster of symptoms including mental confusion, memory loss, and poor muscle control over arms and legs.

Why you need it: thiamin helps the body release energy from carbohydrate foods during metabolism, helps nervous system functioning, and keeps mucous membranes healthy.

For optimal health: 1.5 mg/day of thiamin (those on high-carbohydrate diets may need more)

Best natural food sources: ham, pork, pompano fish, and sunflower seeds

Fortified foods: bread, pasta, rice, ready-to-eat cereals, and regular or quick-cooking hot cereals

Minimum toxic dose: 300 mg/day of thiamin or more may cause drowsiness or a hypersensitive reaction resembling anaphylactic shock.

Selected Studies

Thiamin deficiency may occur in many people with congestive heart failure who are taking diuretic medications. Diuretics that inhibit sodium and chloride reabsorption may lead to deficiencies that in turn contribute to an increased risk of heart failure (*Journal of the American Dietetic Association*, May 1995). If you take diuretics regularly for heart problems, have your thiamin levels checked at least once a year.

Riboflavin—Vitamin B$_2$

Luminous yellow-green color patterns that shimmer in milk whey, liver, and eggs are what first attracted scientists to investigate what was later called riboflavin (RYE-boe-flay-vin). View your eggs or milk at just the right angle and you, too, can see the glorious rainbow of colors.

If you eat lots of overly refined foods, you may not get enough riboflavin. The most common symptoms of riboflavin deficiency include inflammation of the mouth and tongue. Small cracks and fissures at the corners of your mouth may also be a telltale sign that you're not eating right.

Unlike most other water-soluble nutrients, riboflavin is not overly sensitive to high temperatures. The riboflavin in milk can easily withstand pasteurization temperatures. On the other hand, riboflavin is very fragile when exposed to light. That's why milk is packed in paper or plastic containers (not glass). Opaque milk cartons help shield riboflavin from light at the grocery store and in your refrigerator.

Why you need it: riboflavin helps the release of energy from protein, carbohydrate, and fat during metabolism. Promotes normal growth and helps convert the amino acid tryptophan to niacin.

For optimal health: 1.8 mg/day of riboflavin

Best natural food sources: low-fat or nonfat milk and yogurt, and buttermilk (note: the lower the fat content, the higher the riboflavin content of dairy products)

Fortified foods: bread, pasta, and ready-to-eat cereals

Minimum toxic dose: 1 gm/day of riboflavin or more may cause dark urine, nausea, or vomiting

Selected Studies
- A study of fifty-four people with severe migraines were given either 400 mg of riboflavin daily or a placebo. After three months the riboflavin takers had 37 percent fewer migraines (*Neurology,* February 1998). Tell your doctor if you plan to increase your intake of riboflavin to control migraine headaches. There is no information on the long-term effects of high levels of riboflavin.
- Riboflavin deficiency in people with rheumatoid arthritis appears to be linked with continuing inflammation of the joints (*Annals of Rheumatic Disease,* November 1996). People with severe, inflammatory rheumatoid arthritis should evaluate the amount of riboflavin in their diet. If levels are low, higher intakes may help reduce symptoms.

Niacin—B$_3$

Niacin (NYE-a-sin) can be formed in the body from tryptophan, an essential amino acid. Tryptophan is found in meat, poultry, fish, and eggs.

During the depression years, these foods were scarce. Dementia (loss or decrease in mental function), diarrhea, and dermatitis are the three Ds of niacin deficiency, also known as pellagra. When corn became a staple food in the early 1700s in Europe, pellagra reached epidemic proportions. Reliance on corn foods in the southeastern United States in the early 1900s sparked our own pellagra epidemic. That's because the niacin in corn is bound to a protein molecule that prevents absorption. In 1941 the federal grain enrichment program was developed as a response to the devastation caused by pellagra. Today, many corn-based products like tortillas are soaked in lime water, which releases the niacin and makes it usable. Our higher standard of living and the increased availability of protein-rich foods has all but eliminated pellagra.

Niacin can lower blood cholesterol in certain people, when taken in very high amounts. Remember that megadoses of a vitamin change the way that these nutrients work in your body. Niacin in megadose amounts acts like many cholesterol-lowering drugs. A common side effect from niacin therapy is skin flushing. Time-release niacin supplements were developed to help reduce this effect, but these slow-absorbing formulas have been found to be more toxic to the liver. If you have liver disease, gout, peptic ulcers, or a high intake of alcohol, regular and time-release niacin supplements are not recommended.

Why you need it: niacin helps the release of energy from protein, carbohydrate, and fat during metabolism; maintains normal function of skin, nerves, and digestive system.

For optimal health: 14 mg/day of niacin

Best natural food sources: chicken, lamb, pork, veal, mackerel, mullet, salmon, swordfish

Fortified foods: breads, pasta, and cereal

Minimum toxic dose: Amounts as low as 50 mg/day of niacin can produce flushing if taken on an empty stomach. 500 mg or more may cause high blood sugar, itching, irregular heart rhythm, nausea, and ulcers. Blurred vision, eye and eyelid swelling, and loss of eyebrows and eyelashes are also common side effects of too much niacin.

Selected Studies

A study of the side effects of niacin drug therapy when used to lower cholesterol showed a variety of problems. Heart palpitations; worsening of diabetic control; and accelerated peptic ulcer, gout, and hepatitis disease were common (*Coronary Artery Disease*, April 1996). Niacin therapy should be used only in people with significantly high blood cholesterol levels. Don't take niacin in large amounts without medical guidance.

Pyridoxine—Vitamin B$_6$

Pyridoxine's (peer-i-DOX-een) claim to fame came in the early 1980s when it was proclaimed the premenstrual syndrome (PMS) vitamin. It didn't take long—just until 1983—to see the first descriptions of toxicity described in the *New England Journal of Medicine* (see Selected Studies, below). Even today, many physicians and clinics that specialize in treating PMS routinely prescribe between 800 and 2,000 mg of B$_6$ per day.

The most important function of vitamin B$_6$ is protein metabolism. It helps cells figure out which amino acids to break down for energy and which to convert into other amino acids. It's also crucial in making key nervous system regulators or neurotransmitters. It's the link between B$_6$ and neurotransmitters that started the PMS research.

Why you need it: vitamin B$_6$ helps use protein to build body tissue, aids in metabolism of fat, maintains chemical balance of body fluids, and regulates water excretion. The higher your protein intake, the higher your need is for vitamin B$_6$.

For optimal health: 1.3 mg/day of B$_6$

Best natural food sources: bananas, plantain, and chicken

Fortified foods: ready-to-eat cereals and oatmeal

Minimum toxic dose: 200 mg/day of vitamin B$_6$ or more over time may cause physiological dependence, which leads to undesirable higher needs. 500 mg or more may cause nerve disorders, pain, numbness, sun-induced skin rash, or weakness in limbs. May cause depression when large amounts are taken with oral contraceptives.

Selected Studies

- A study published in 1983 first identified the syndrome caused by megadoses of pyridoxine, vitamin B$_6$. Seven individuals taking 2 gm or more of the supplement daily had difficulty walking, numb feet, numbness and clumsiness in the hands, and severely impaired sensation of touch and temperature in both upper and lower limbs. All improved after withdrawal of the supplement (*New England Journal of Medicine,* August 1983). Two gm of B$_6$ is a huge increase over normal needs for this nutrient.

- A study of women and B$_6$ supplementation for PMS found that 100 to 150 mg/day did not show toxic effects. But 500 to 5,000 mg/day in PMS subjects frequently caused serious nerve damage within three years (*Annals of New York Academy of Science,* vol. 588, 1990). The side effects of B$_6$ in megadoses are not worth the modest reduction in PMS symptoms.

Cobalamin—Vitamin B$_{12}$

Cobalamin (ko-BALL-ah-men) can sometimes be a true miracle cure. Picture an elderly woman admitted to the hospital with symptoms of senility.

She is frail, but is able to care for herself, carry on intelligent conversations, and answer common questions. Gradually her mental abilities fade to the point that Alzheimer's or senility are considered. After ruling out these and other serious problems, a simple injection of vitamin B_{12} leads to sudden, dramatic improvements. She's up, walking the halls of her hospital wing, smiling, and is back to normal.

Getting enough vitamin B_{12} can be a problem for many older adults because aging bodies don't secrete the amount of stomach acid necessary for absorption of the vitamin. A B_{12} deficiency can cause serious neuralgic problems. Low levels may also increase susceptibility to heart attack and stroke. Folic acid and B_{12} work together. If there is too much folic acid, a deficiency of B_{12} can be hidden from routine blood analyses. Vegans and other vegetarians who eat almost no animal foods may develop a deficiency in vitamin B_{12} over time. Have your blood level of vitamin B_{12} checked about every five years if you don't eat meat, fish, poultry, eggs, and milk.

Why you need it: vitamin B_{12} is essential to help fight certain cancers, cardiovascular disease, depression, and mental dysfunction. Vitamin B_{12} works with folate to make red blood cells. It also serves in every body cell as a vital part of many body chemicals, and helps the body use fatty acids and some amino acids.

Optimal intake: 2.5 to 3 mcg/day of B_6

Best natural food sources: meat, fish, poultry, eggs, and milk

Fortified foods: cereals and breads

Minimum toxic level: none known

Folate

Folate (FOE-late), folic (FOLL-ick) acid, folacin (FOE-la-cin)—whatever you choose to call it—has earned the honor of contributing the most striking public health improvement of any vitamin this decade. Optimal amounts of folic acid during conception and early fetal development drastically reduce the chances of having a baby born with a devastating neural tube defect (NTD) like spina bifida. Before the link with folate was discovered, about 2,500 babies were born with NTDs in the United States each year. When more women start consuming the new recommended folate levels, those numbers are expected to drop by half.

Now folate may shine in the spotlight again. Evidence is mounting that optimal levels of folate (along with B_6 and B_{12}) help reduce heart disease by controlling the amount of the amino acid homocysteine (ho-mo-SIS-teen). Normally, homocysteine is converted into other amino acids. If this conversion does not take place fast enough, bloodstream levels of homocysteine become too high. Recent studies show that high levels of homocysteine can damage artery walls, which propels the buildup of atherosclerotic plaque.

Unfortunately, as many as 88 percent of all American fall short when it comes to meeting the DV for this nutrient. Many foods are good sources of folic acid, but you need to eat at least five to nine servings of fruits and vegetables a day to even come close. In fact, folic acid deficiency is the most common vitamin deficiency in the world. Since January 1998, all U.S. manufacturers of enriched products including white flour, white bread, white rice, regular pasta, and hot cereals were required to add folic acid. This fortification adds about 100 to 200 extra mg of folic acid to your daily total. If you typically choose whole wheat-bread, whole-wheat pasta, or brown rice, check the ingredient label to see if folic acid has been added. Fortification is optional for whole-grain products.

Considering the strong evidence that folic acid helps prevent birth defects—not to mention heart disease and possibly cancer—the U.S. Public Health Service advises every woman of childbearing age to consume 0.4 mg each day. Most multivitamins supply that amount of folic acid, which is also available as a separate supplement.

Why you need it: folate helps to form red blood cells, forms the genetic material (DNA and RNA) within each cell, and functions as part of coenzymes in amino acid formation.

For optimal health: 400 to 600 mcg/day of folate from a synthetic supplement, plus food sources; the higher level for any woman who might get pregnant and all pregnant women during their first trimester. Older people with reduced stomach acid have less absorption and therefore need more.

Best natural food sources: spinach (cooked), black-eyed peas, kidney beans, pinto beans, lentils, oatmeal, asparagus, and orange juice

Fortified foods: bread, pasta, rice, and ready-to-eat hot and cold cereals

Minimum toxic dose: 1,000 mcg (1 gm) or more may hide a vitamin B_{12} deficiency, decrease zinc absorption, and produce damaging folacin crystals in the kidneys. Amounts over 1,500 mcg can cause decreased appetite, abdominal bloating, flatulence, nausea, and interference with anticonvulsant drugs used to prevent seizures.

Selected Studies

- A meta-analysis of twelve randomized controlled trials that assessed the effects of folic acid supplements on blood homocysteine concentrations found that dietary folic acid reduced blood homocysteine concentrations in those with elevated levels by 25 percent in the range of 0.5 to 5 mg folic acid daily. Vitamin B_{12} supplementation of 0.5 mg daily produced an additional 7 percent reduction in blood homocysteine (*British Medical Journal*, 1998).

- A study of seventy-five men and women showed that folic acid intakes of 500 to 665 mcg per day increased red-cell folic acid levels and decreased harmful homocysteine blood levels, thereby reducing the risk of heart disease (*New England Journal of Medicine*, April 1998).

- A three-month study showed that women who increased their intake of foods rich in folic acid had significantly less red-cell folate levels compared to women who received supplements. Women who either took supplements or ate folate-fortified foods were the only ones who improved their folate status (*Lancet*, May 1996). It may be unreasonable to expect women of childbearing age to get the recommended amount of folate from foods alone. If you are of childbearing age, you should be taking folate supplements.

- Two studies, one of 5,000 Canadians and one of 80,000 U.S. nurses, found those who reported eating diets high in folate had a lower risk of heart disease over the following fifteen years (*Journal of the American Medical Association*, June 1996, and *Journal of the American Medical Association*, August 1998).

Biotin

Bios is the Greek word for life. Bacteria in the intestines usually produce enough biotin (BYE-oh-tin), but it is widely available in common foods. Biotin is best known as an essential nutrient for keeping your hair and skin healthy.

If you know someone who likes to eat raw eggs, here's some trivia to convince them to stop. In addition to risking serious food-borne disease, people who consume huge quantities of raw egg whites (fifteen or more per day) get too much of a substance called avidin that prevents the absorption of biotin. Most adults have the right mix of intestinal bacteria to produce their own biotin. But anyone on long-term anticonvulsant drugs, which can inhibit biotin uptake, are at risk for deficiency.

Why you need it: biotin helps the release of energy from protein, carbohydrate, and fat during metabolism. It also helps strengthen hair and nails.

For optimal health: 25 to 35 mcg/day of biotin

Best natural food sources: eggs, liver, and yeast breads

Fortified foods: ready-to-eat hot and cold cereals

Minimum toxic dose: none known

Selected Studies

- At the University of Ferrara, Italy, it was discovered that biotin deficiency may be associated with epileptic and/or convulsive disorders (*Neuroreport*, May 1996). Biotin, or any other nutrient, cannot cure any disease such as epilepsy. If you are at risk for seizures, be sure you eat plenty of foods rich in this nutrient.

- A study concluded that biotin excretion may increase during pregnancy, making biotin levels in the body decrease as a pregnancy progresses to the latter stages (*Journal of Nutrition*, vol. 127, 1997). Maintaining biotin level is another important reason to continue taking prenatal vitamin and mineral supplements during your entire pregnancy.

Pantothenic Acid

Pantothenic (pan-toe-THIN-ick) acid gets around, but it's not a popular nutrient. The proof is on the food label. Scan the nutrition facts panel of your favorite fortified foods and you won't find pantothenic acid listed along with the other B vitamins routinely added. That's because pantothenic acid deficiency is so rare we don't even know what it might look like. *Pantos,* a Greek root word, means "everywhere." Almost every food you eat contains some pantothenic acid. But that's just half the story.

If you rely on heavily processed, nutrient-fortified foods to provide your vitamin and mineral needs, you can end up with suboptimal nutrient levels. The pantothenic acid that occurs naturally in foods is significantly destroyed during food processing. If you don't eat a wide variety of unprocessed foods, you will fall short on pantothenic acid at the same time your intake of other nutrients looks good. For example, some women who eat a minimal amount of calories trying to control their weight often choose highly processed fortified foods that appear to be nutritious (like breakfast cereals and fruit-granola bars). They often have a salad or small meal and then add in fat-free chips or cookies and diet soft drinks. It's startling to see their nutrient intakes showing well over 100 percent of the RDA for popular vitamins and minerals. In contrast, they consume just 50 to 75 percent of the RDA for nutrients like pantothenic acid that are supposed to be so easy to get.

Why you need it: pantothenic acid helps release of energy from protein, carbohydrate, and fat during metabolism; maintains blood sugar levels; aids in the forming of red blood cells, hormones, and substances needed for nerve transmission.

For optimal health: 5 to 10 mg/day of pantothenic acid; athletes, those who perform vigorous manual work, and pregnant women need the higher amounts.

Best natural food sources: almost all natural foods

Fortified foods: whole-grain cereals

Minimum toxic dose: 10,000 mg/day of pantothenic acid or more may cause diarrhea or water retention

Selected Studies

■ Early investigation suggests that pantothenic acid and its derivatives appear to protect against damage done to cells by oxygen free radicals by increasing levels of the compound CoA (coenzyme A) (*Free Radical Biology Medicine,* December 1995).

■ It is hypothesized that pantothenic acid deficiency may cause the onset of acne, and that a cure for acne would be to supplement the acne sufferer with liberal amounts of pantothenic acid (*Medical Hypotheses,* June 1995). This research just identified an area for future clinical study and offers no proof at this time.

Vitamin C

Millions of people religiously swallow supplements of vitamin C (sometimes referred to as ascorbic acid) hoping to cure everything from the common cold to cancer. There's lots of fiction surrounding vitamin C; here are the facts. Vitamin C:

■ prevents scurvy, a disease reported to have caused the deaths of onehalf to two-thirds of all sailors on extended sea voyages from the sixteenth to eighteenth centuries. Scurvy is still a common affliction in undeveloped countries with deficient food supplies.

■ stimulates antibodies that help fight infection and illness

■ helps stop the production of cancer-causing nitrosamines in the stomach

■ helps improve the body's ability to use folic acid and iron

■ helps to rid the body of toxic levels of stored lead

■ prevents free radical damage, which leads to cancer and promotes tumor growth, by working as an antioxidant

■ is harmful to tooth enamel when chewable forms are taken daily

■ is needed in higher than normal amounts by smokers and people who take oral contraceptives, anticoagulants, aspirin products, sulfa drugs, or tetracycline

■ in large amounts can cause false negative tests for diabetes (urine) and colon cancer (fecal occult blood)

With all due respect to Nobel prize–winning scientist and vitamin C advocate Dr. Linus Pauling, over thirty years of research shows no clear evidence that large intakes of vitamin C can prevent or cure colds. What it can do is prevent scurvy, which usually first shows up as cracked and bleeding gums. British sailors were nicknamed limeys because of the limes, lemons, and other citrus fruits that were provided to prevent scurvy during long seas voyages.

Vitamin C is a puzzling nutrient. Only humans, monkeys, guinea pigs, a few birds, and some fish need vitamin C from foods. Every other living thing makes its own C from the sugar glucose. The same amount of vitamin C that prevents scurvy (10 mg) is not the same amount that can produce optimal health. Your body becomes saturated with vitamin C at intakes between 200 and 250 milligrams. If you take too much vitamin C, it stays in your small intestine and attracts water, which will eventually cause diarrhea.

Why you need it: vitamin C forms collagen (connective tissue); maintains capillaries, bones, and teeth; aids wound healing; and increases iron absorption. As an antioxidant, it prevents cell damage and can help stop the production of cancer-causing nitrosamines in the stomach.

For optimal health: 200 mg/day of vitamin C

Best natural food sources: fruits—cantaloupe, grapefruit, grapefruit juice, honeydew, kiwi, mango, oranges, orange juice, papaya, pineapple juice, raspberries, strawberries, tangelo, tangerine, watermelon; vegetables— asparagus, broccoli, brussels sprouts, cabbage, cauliflower, kale, kohlrabi, mustard greens, peppers, plantain, potato (with skin), rutabagas, snow peas, sweet potato, tomato, tomato juice or sauce

Fortified foods: some juice and juice drinks and ready-to-eat cereals

Minimum toxic dose: 500 to 1,000 mg/day of vitamin C or more may cause diarrhea, headache, and cramping. Large doses over time may cause urinary tract infection, kidney stones in people with kidney disease, and erosion of tooth enamel (with chewable vitamin C).

Selected Studies

■ The National Academy of Sciences reports a study of seven young men who were kept in a hospital to closely monitor their food intake. They were fed diets without vitamin C and then given supplements ranging from 30 mg to 2,500 mg of vitamin C. At an intake of 200 mg per day, researchers found that both the immune cells and blood were saturated with C; amounts above this did not result in higher retention of the nutrient (*Proceedings from the National Academy of Sciences,* 1996). There is no known benefit to intakes above 200 mg of vitamin C.

■ A University of California research team using data from the National Health Survey of nine thousand people aged 20 to 74 found that women with high blood levels of vitamin C developed half as many gallstones as those with moderate intakes. Vitamin C increases the enzyme activity that converts cholesterol to bile.

- A meta-analysis of the six largest vitamin C supplementation (over 1,000 mg/day) studies, including over five thousand episodes in all, has been analyzed, and it is shown that common cold incidence is not reduced in the vitamin C–supplemented groups compared with the placebo groups. However, in four studies of British schoolboys with chronically poor vitamin C status, a highly significant reduction in common cold incidence was found when they were given supplements (*British Journal of Nutrition,* January 1997). Vitamin C in megadoses does not prevent or reduce the number of colds you will get. If you are deficient in vitamin C, increasing your intake will help strengthen your immune system.

- A report of an expert review panel from the National Institutes of Health recommends that a new RDA value for vitamin C be updated to between 120 and 200 mg/day. They emphasized that whenever possible, the vitamin C should come from fruits and vegetables, and that people can get the recommended amount by eating five servings of these foods daily (*Journal of the American Medical Association,* April 1999). See our list of foods high in vitamin C on the preceding page. A diet rich in fruits and vegetables may also be beneficial in helping to prevent some types of cancer.

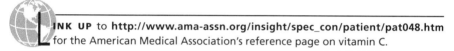

LINK UP to http://www.ama-assn.org/insight/spec_con/patient/pat048.htm for the American Medical Association's reference page on vitamin C.

VITAMIN-LIKE COMPOUNDS

They don't have the status of a full-fledged vitamin, but the following vitamin-like compounds are important. Included are a variety of compounds that are necessary for metabolism. There are no RDA or DV for these nutrients. Most of these compounds are found in animal foods. Because vegans (who eat no animal products) have never been shown to have deficiencies, it appears clear that your body makes all you need. Premature infants, though, may need an outside source of choline, carnitine, and taurine. Their bodies are not developed enough to make these substances on their own. Breast milk is loaded with these compounds, but many tiny premature babies aren't able to breast-feed or be given breast milk.

Healthy adults use amino acids and glucose to make these substances. If you have a debilitating disease, eating more foods high in these nutrients may be important. Here's a brief description of what we know about them.

Choline

Do you have a good memory? Perhaps you should thank choline (KO-leen). It helps your brain store memories and keeps your emotions and judgment in line. Without choline you'd be a forgetful, irrational, emotional mess (or just more so). It's a precursor to the nerve messenger acetylcholine. It's also a type of fat that maintains smooth, fluid connections between brain cells.

One form of this fat, phosphatidyl choline, is the active ingredient in lecithin. Most people consume about 1,000 mg of lecithin from foods as part of a normal diet.

The Food and Nutrition Board recently set a precedent by classifying choline as a nutrient, even though it's not required by all groups of the population. The new recommendation for choline is 500 mg per day. Research suggests that only men and pregnant or breast-feeding women require a dietary source of choline.

Some forms of supplemental choline, such as choline bitartrate or choline chloride, can cause a fishy body odor. Other side effects from supplements include stomach and intestinal distress, loss of appetite, vomiting, nausea, and diarrhea. Some researchers believe that high doses of choline may increase the risk of stomach cancer. That's because choline can transform compounds in ways that cause them to develop into carcinogenic nitrosamines.

Pregnant women have lots of choline circulating around the placenta. That's the organ that passes nutrients from the mother to the developing baby. It' been suggested that since choline is important for fetal growth, it must have magic properties that are helpful in growing new tissue. No research has made the connection.

Selected Studies
Choline circulating into the brain decreases with age. Because choline plays a key role in the structure and function of brain neurons, this change may contribute to the onset of brain impairments during aging (*Journal of the American Medical Association*, September 1995).

Carnitine
Acetyl L-carnitine (ah-SEE-tull el-KAR-nah-teen) is a molecule that helps transport fat into the mitochondria of your cells. Mitochondria are tiny energy factories in each living cell. Carnitine is a substance your body supplies for you, as long as you have enough vitamins B_1, B_6, iron, and lysine to make it yourself. Vegetarians might have low levels of carnitine if their diets are low in lysine. Such a deficiency is possible because lysine is found in high concentrations in muscle tissue; if you don't eat meat, you might not get enough.

Carnitine is also popular with body-builders, who believe it helps them add muscle bulk and improve endurance. No evidence for these claims has been documented. Many supplement manufacturers have jumped into the market with their own versions of carnitine. The National Organization for Rare Disorders tested twelve brands of L-carnitine to see just how truthful the label claims were. L-carnitine is a supplement critical to people with a particularly deadly form of genetic carnitine deficiency.

Many of the brands tested showed a wide variation in L-carnitine among the individual pills sold in the same bottle. Pills in one brand ranged from 20 to 85 percent of the amount that was stated on the label. Two brands didn't even contain any detectable carnitine.

Inositol

If you want to keep from losing your money as well as your hair, don't buy inositol (in-AH-seh-tall). Touted as a treatment for everything from hair loss to weight control, inositol does have a redeeming role as a supplement. It keeps membranes healthy and shuttles needed fat from place to place. It helps keep your bone marrow, eye tissue, and intestines in good condition.

Premature infants and diabetics have the biggest chance of not having enough of this vitamin-like substance. Some research shows that diabetics with low levels of inositol in their nerve tissue may benefit from extra inositol, which might decrease the nerve damage, a complication common with diabetes.

Taurine

Taurine (TAR-een) is a sulfur-containing nutrient that helps manage your nervous system by keeping your nerves and muscles working together smoothly. Most taurine is found in your heart and other muscles, white blood cells, and central nervous system. It also is part of the bile that is used to help digest fats and absorb fat-soluble vitamins. It's surprising that little taurine is found in animal products since muscle is a main active storage site in humans. Taurine is one of the nutrients that your body can make itself if you have enough protein and vitamin B_6.

INK UP to http://www.nutrition.about.com/library/blmicronutrients.htm for a complete reference of each vitamin.

PILLS IN FOOD FORM

So, just how much of what do you need? Before you dash to the nearest supplement counter, take stock of what you are already adding to your foods in terms of extra vitamins and minerals. You may be swallowing a supplement without realizing it. Some foods are required by law to be enriched or fortified with additional nutrients. Milk and other dairy products have added vitamins A and D. One 8-ounce glass of milk provides 100 IU of vitamin D and 500 IU of vitamin A. Many grains like bread, rice, and pasta have added B vitamins, iron, and folate.

Food companies also voluntarily add nutrients to foods to increase their marketing appeal. Several leading cereal companies spray on between

25 and 100 percent of the DV of selected nutrients. Compare cereal nutrition fact labels the next time you are in the grocery store and you'll notice the randomness of how nutrients are added to foods. Eating a serving of cereal poured from one of these packages is like taking a supplement, but only if you drink the milk in the bottom of the bowl, since that's where most of the added water-soluble vitamins end up. Keep in mind that there are more than forty known nutrients and only a few of these are added to any one food. The helter-skelter way nutrients are pumped into food can skew well-intentioned food choices. You might gobble up plenty of the popular nutrients that are cheap or in vogue and still be deficient in those that are too expensive or unpopular with food manufacturers.

As long as a "food" meets the minimum requirements for certain nutrients, it can replace a real fruit, vegetable, or grain, according to current USDA school lunch standards. Fortified candy and doctored-up sugary beverages are standing in for more nutritious foods in lunchrooms across the country. No matter what the guidelines say, vitamin-laced gummy candies are not the nutritional equivalent of a serving of fruit. Orange juice is far superior to an orange drink fortified with added vitamin C. Fortified beverages usually lack essentials including folic acid, vitamin A, potassium, phosphorus, and even a little fiber found in 100 percent juice.

Advertising campaigns encourage on-the-go yuppies, baby boomers, and their aging parents to get a "boost" from a can of fortified imitation milk-like beverages such as Ensure or Slim Fast. There are a wide variety of fortified candy and granola bars, milkshakes, puddings, soups, and cookies marketed as total meal replacements. Where are you supposed to get fiber? What about other nutrients? How about satisfaction from eating flavorful food? Food is more than just something to swallow on your way out the door—it's meant to be savored and enjoyed. A diet of vitamin-mineral fortified food fragments can't begin to compare with the health benefits and emotional satisfaction from eating a variety of fresh, wholesome, and delicious foods. Special nutritional supplements do have a place for individuals with severe health problems like cancer or cystic fibrosis, but they can't stand in for more healthful meals and snacks.

It's critical to keep in perspective the fact that nutrient requirements are interrelated. You need appropriate amounts of all nutrients to optimize your health. Meeting your nutrient needs by relying on the selected supplements included in fortified foods almost ensures you will not be eating well. Variety in food selection is what promotes optimal nutrition.

A daily multiple vitamin-mineral product that provides 100 percent of the RDA is a good place to start. Choose one with as many essential nutrients as possible. Some one-a-day–type brands have fewer than ten nutrients; others more than two dozen.

If you have a specific lifestyle or health-related condition, your need for a particular nutrient or group of nutrients may be increased. For example:

- Most women and girls don't eat enough calories to be able to meet their iron needs.
- Cigarette smokers need double the usual amount of vitamin C.
- Women on oral contraceptives have an increased need for B vitamins and vitamin C.
- Prolonged use of antibiotics can alter intestinal bacteria that normally help to manufacture B vitamins and vitamin K.
- The elderly tend to absorb less vitamin B_{12}, D, and C.
- Individuals with broken bones, recovering from surgery, or body burns need increased amounts of most nutrients, especially vitamin C and calcium if movement is restricted.
- Heavy alcohol users frequently have elevated nutrient losses associated with diarrhea and increased urine output and require both vitamin and mineral supplementation.
- Many medications can cause a deficiency of particular vitamins and minerals. Always ask your doctor or pharmacist for drug-nutrient interactions when you begin a new prescription or over-the-counter medication.

THE BOTTOM LINE

Carefully selected supplements may benefit most people. A multiple vitamin/mineral supplement is a good start. If you don't drink milk, you might need additional calcium. Research is confirming that vitamin E, in amounts higher than you can get from foods, offers protective benefits. But don't misinterpret the message. Popping a pill doesn't mean you can forget about selecting a variety of wholesome foods. While this book reviews the optimal amounts of vitamins and minerals, it does not suggest that supplementation is the preferred way to get them. Evidence that supplements help prevent or fight disease pales next to data that show the positive effects of eating foods, especially fruits and vegetables.

Eat the most healthful way you can, and then determine what might need improvement based on your individual circumstances. Remember, vitamin and mineral supplements are not magic pills; nor will they neutralize a high-fat, low-fiber diet of processed foods. Don't rely on supplements as a nutritional shortcut—you won't come out a winner. People of different ages, genders, and health statuses have different nutritional needs. What supplements should you take? We'll summarize that at the end of the next chapter on minerals.

Vitamin Needs for Special Situations

Nutrient	Highest Federal Standard (RDA or DV)	Optimal Intake	Individuals with Special Needs*
Vitamin A	1,000 RE (retinol equivalents)	5,000 IU	Diabetics and people who are exposed to toxic chemicals at work or heavy air pollution where they live
Vitamin C	60 mg	200–500 mg	Women on oral contraceptives and all smokers
Vitamin D	5–15 mcg	10–15 mcg	Sun-avoiders, people over 70, some vegetarians, and people with kidney failure
Vitamin E	8–10 mg	50–200 IU	Those over 55 and people with hyperthyroiditis
Vitamin K	60–80 mcg	65–200 mg	People on very low-calorie diets
Thiamin	1–1.5 mg	Not known	People over 70, heavy coffee and tea drinkers, and those on very low-calorie or high-carbohydrate diets
Riboflavin	1.2–1.7 mg	Not known	People who eat lots of processed foods, very active adults, those with low calcium intakes, and individuals with low thyroid disorders
Niacin	13–19 mg	Not known	People over 55, diabetics, very active individuals, and those with hyperthyroid disorders
Vitamin B_6	1.4–2 mg	Not known	Women on oral contraceptives
Folate	200 mcg	400–600 mcg	People over 70, women on oral contraceptives, all women who could become pregnant, and people with sickle cell anemia
Vitamin B_{12}	2 mcg	Not known	Vegans
Biotin	100 mcg	Not known	Those on antibiotics, smokers, and women on oral contraceptives
Pantothenic Acid	7 mg	5–12 mg	People over 55, those on very low-calorie diets, and smokers

* Pregnant and breast-feeding women, alcoholics, and drug abusers have increased needs for most nutrients.

6

Minerals

Minerals are inorganic chemicals; that is, they are not attached to a carbon atom. They aid many biochemical functions necessary for growth, development, and overall health. Like vitamins, many minerals are a part of enzymes. Minerals are the catalysts that help enzymes to operate. Different minerals are critical to enzyme systems either because they are part of the enzyme itself or because they help the enzyme to work properly. We each need more than 100 milligrams (mg) of minerals daily. An adult male stores about 5 pounds of minerals throughout his body.

There are several classifications for dietary minerals depending on the function they serve and how much you need. They are:

- major minerals—minerals of which you need more than 250 mg per day. Calcium is a major mineral, needed in amounts ranging from 800 to 1,500 mg per day.
- electrolytes—minerals that dissolve in water.
- trace elements—minerals you need in very tiny amounts, less than 20 mg per day. Iron is a trace element; most people require just 10 to 18 mg daily.
- heavy metals—toxic minerals that even in minute amounts can cause harm. They include aluminum, arsenic, cadmium, lead, and mercury.

Zinc, copper, iron, and other minerals are deposited in earth and rock. They find their way into foods because plant roots absorb minerals from dirt and water. Red meat is the best food source of minerals because an animal will consume vast amounts of plants over its lifetime. The minerals from plants are concentrated in the animal's tissues. Whole grains are the best nonmeat mineral source, followed by fruits and vegetables.

COLLOIDAL CONFUSION

Colloidal minerals are tiny particles suspended in a liquid with a yellow tint. It's the yellow color that indicates the presence of dissolved organic matter. Promoters of colloidal minerals claim that the suspension helps to improve absorption. However, there is absolutely no scientific proof for this hypothesis. If you choose to take the expensive colloidal preparations commonly available, beware of their potential toxic risk. Although concentrations of hazardous substances may be low, long-term exposure can result in a buildup of exotic and dangerous minerals including lead, arsenic, aluminum, mercury, iridium, and rhodium.

GET THE LEAD OUT

What do paint, pencils, pollution, pipes, and pottery have in common? They can all contain traces of the toxic mineral lead. Too much lead in your system can lead to erratic behavior and mental retardation. In fact, some historians think the fall of the Roman empire was a result of chronic lead poisoning from drinking wine and eating food from vessels loaded with lead.

MAJOR MINERALS

Calcium

The message to get enough calcium has saturated just about every medium except our bodies. Bone is a growing tissue that is constantly being broken down and rebuilt, just like your hair and nails. About 20 percent of your skeleton is made brand new every year. Calcium intake is critical because it's the most abundant mineral in your body, and one of the most essential.

Women in their 20s start to lose bone mass—it's one of those inevitable parts of getting older. Since it takes men's bodies longer to mature to begin with, they start depleting bone mass a little later than women. More women die each year from hip fractures related to osteoporosis than from breast cancer, uterine cancer, and ovarian cancer combined.

Why you need it: calcium builds bone and teeth and maintains their strength; assists in muscle contraction, blood clotting, and maintenance of cell membranes. The connection between calcium intake and osteoporosis prevention is so strong that the Food and Drug Administration (FDA) has ruled that food labels can advertise the link. Calcium is too bulky to include at high enough levels in multivitamin tablets, so separate supplements are usually required for those who need significant extra calcium. The National Osteoporosis Foundation recommends 1,200 to 1,500 mg of calcium per day for females ages 11 to 24, 1,000 mg per day for women age 25 and over, 1,500 mg daily for postmenopausal women not taking estrogen, and 1,200 to 1,500 mg of calcium daily for pregnant or lactating women.

For optimal health: 1,000 to 1,500 mg/day of calcium

Best natural food sources: cheese, milk, and yogurt

Fortified foods: orange juice, rice, and tofu (made with calcium sulfate)

Minimum toxic dose: 2,500 mg/day of calcium or more may cause nausea; vomiting; low blood pressure; irregular heartbeat; kidney stones; impaired absorption of iron, zinc, and magnesium.

How Much Calcium in My Supplement?

All calcium supplements don't provide equal amounts of absorbable calcium. The lower the absorption rate, the more you need to take to get an adequate supply. Never take bone meal, oyster shell, or dolomite; these supplements can contain lead and other toxic metals.

Type of Calcium	% Absorption
Calcium citrate	74%
Calcium carbonate	40%
Calcium phosphate	32%
Calcium lactate	18%
Calcium gluconate	9%

Source: Adapted from the *Journal of Bone Mineral Research,* 1989

Selected Studies
- A meta-analysis of fourteen studies found that adding 300 mg of calcium daily in the form of supplements or the equivalent of one 8-ounce glass of milk decreased bone fractures in susceptible populations from 25 percent to 70 percent (*Journal of Bone Mineral Research,* September 1997). These results were likely to be an underestimate of calcium's true effect because of inaccurate measurement of dietary calcium in the observational studies, said researchers.

- This meta-analysis of calcium studies and blood pressure reviewed fifty-six articles involving a total of 2,421 research subjects. Researchers found that calcium supplementation may lead to a small reduction in systolic (the first number, e.g., **120/80**) blood pressure (*Journal of the American Medical*

Association, April 1996). This study zeroed in on calcium supplements. Later studies show that dietary calcium does have an impact on lowering blood pressure.

Magnesium

A special region in Greece, Magnesia, was frequently visited in ancient times because of the magical powers within a salty, white powder. Ever heard of "Milk of Magnesia"? Magnesium works as an antacid in small doses and as a laxative in large amounts. This multipurpose mineral is also what early photographers used to create light flashes before the days of flash cubes or electronic flashes.

Magnesium is the trigger that activates over 300 enzymes. Enzymes regulate many body functions, including energy production and muscle contractions. Magnesium works as a signal for muscles to contract and relax; when the muscles that line major blood vessels contract, it impacts your blood pressure. Magnesium helps just about every other chemical in your body do its job.

Since the 1960s, researchers have known that people who live in areas where the water is "hard" often have lower rates of heart disease and stroke. ("Hard" water contains more calcium, magnesium, and other minerals than "soft" water.) But the amount of magnesium in hard water is typically no more than 3 to 20 mg per liter—less than 10 percent of what people get from a day's intake of food.

Why you need it: magnesium builds bones, forms proteins, helps release energy stored in muscles, and regulates body temperature.

For optimal health: 300 to 500 mg/day of magnesium

Best natural food sources: no food provides even 25 percent of the RDA in one serving. Foods that provide 10 to 24 percent of the RDA include whole grains, broccoli, spinach, skin-on potatoes, dry beans, dry peas, lentils, nuts, nut butters, pumpkin seeds, nonfat yogurt, and halibut.

Fortified foods: none

Minimum toxic dose: not known, but too much from supplements may cause nausea, vomiting, low blood pressure, muscle weakness, or irregular heartbeat

Selected Studies
- A study of sixteen healthy people who were placed on magnesium-deficient diets became less insulin sensitive. Their insulin became less effective at getting sugar from their blood into their cells. A high percentage of type 2 diabetics have a deficiency of magnesium inside their cells (*Hypertension,*

1993). Insulin sensitivity is one of the first steps that can lead to diabetes. No one knows which comes first—the diabetes or the magnesium deficiency. It's not clear whether magnesium supplements can help diabetes.

■ The Atherosclerosis Risk in Communities Study (ARIC) has been following about fourteen thousand middle-aged people for up to seven years. They found that men and women with the lowest levels of magnesium in their blood at the start of study were twice as likely to be diagnosed later with diabetes as those with the highest levels of magnesium (*Diabetes*, September 1997). Magnesium and insulin need each other. Without magnesium, your pancreas won't secrete enough insulin—or the insulin it secretes won't be efficient enough—to control you blood sugar. And without insulin, magnesium doesn't get transported from your blood into your cells, where it does most of its work.

Phosphorus

Phosphorus is second only to its mineral relative calcium in abundance in your body. Like calcium, phosphorus helps build strong bones and teeth.

Do you consume soft drinks or take antacids that contain aluminum hydroxide? Check the ingredient list. If you find it listed on the label, you might be disrupting your body's delicate calcium/phosphorus balance. Too much aluminum hydroxide may decrease your absorption of phosphorus, and that can lead to weakened bones. Processed foods are another culprit, frequently adding phosphorus-containing preservatives to your diet. Milk provides the best ratio of phosphorus to calcium.

Why you need it: phosphorus builds bone and teeth; helps release energy from protein, fat, and carbohydrates during metabolism; forms genetic material, cell membranes, and many enzymes.

For optimal health: 800 to 1,200 mg/day of phosphorous

Best natural food sources: carp, mackerel, salmon (canned), swordfish, chocolate milk, and low-fat or nonfat yogurt

Fortified foods: none

Minimum toxic dose: 12,000 mg/day of phosphorus or more may cause shortness of breath, irregular heartbeat, or seizures.

ELECTROLYTES

Chloride

You may not know much about chloride alone, but it's part of a famous couple known as table salt (sodium chloride). Adults typically need a minimum of 750 mg of chloride a day. Part of that goes to form hydrochloric acid—better known as stomach acid. This caustic compound is what helps you break down food so individual nutrients can be absorbed and used by the body.

Why you need it: chloride regulates cell fluids, aids the digestion of food, helps nutrient absorption, and helps to transmit nerve impulses.

For optimal health: 750 mg/day (the amount found in ¼ teaspoon of table salt), more if you exercise

Best natural food sources: table salt and salted foods

Fortified foods: none

Minimum toxic dose: not known, but too much may cause weakness, confusion, increased blood pressure, or coma

Potassium

It takes a minimum of 2,000 milligrams of potassium a day to aid digestion and make protein. Potassium is so important to protein that lots of it is stored in your muscles. Often, leg cramps are linked to a potassium deficiency. When your muscles cramp they're screaming "I'm tired, hungry, and need to rest!" Cramps actually force your muscles to remain inactive until they have a chance to recover. Potassium also affects blood pressure by relaxing the artery walls. Relaxed walls allow blood to flow through smoothly, and that helps keep your blood pressure low.

Why you need it: potassium helps muscles to contract; maintains fluid and electrolyte balance; helps send nerve impulses; releases energy from protein, carbohydrates, and fat during metabolism.

For optimal health: 2,000 to 5,000 mg/day of potassium

Best natural food sources: 100 percent bran cereal, apricots (dried), bananas, orange juice, peaches (dried), pomegranate, prunes, prune juice, chard, plantains, potatoes, pumpkin, spinach, squash, tomatoes (cooked), tomato juice, pork, veal, carp, catfish, cod, flounder, mullet, black beans, kidney beans, lima beans, soybeans, lentils, dry peas (cooked), milk, and yogurt

Fortified foods: none

Minimum toxic dose: not established; large amounts of potassium from supplements may cause increased heart rate, low blood pressure, convulsions, paralysis of limbs, or cardiac arrest

Selected Studies
A 1996 Johns Hopkins and National Institutes of Health meta-analyses of thirty-three clinical trials on over 2,600 individuals found that those with high blood pressure who consumed an extra 2,000 mg or more of potassium lowered blood pressure a small but significant amount.

Sodium

Do you reach for the salt shaker as soon as your plate is served? You don't need that extra sodium, but will it harm you? The answer to that questions is still being debated.

If you ate only unprocessed foods and added no table salt, you'd still get enough sodium to meet normal needs. Just 400 to 500 milligrams of sodium is enough to keep your body fluids and blood pressure in balance. Of course, if you are extremely active, have a fever or prolonged diarrhea, or are vomiting you need extra sodium. That's why soup, broth, and saltine crackers are frequently recommended during illness.

Sodium is the nutrient most frequently associated as a villain in blood pressure. High blood pressure, or hypertension, affects about 50 million Americans—one in four adults. It's the leading cause of stroke and contributes to heart attack, heart failure, and kidney failure. Some Americans, including those over 70 and African Americans, have a particularly high risk from high blood pressure.

Sodium is just one factor that may affect blood pressure. Various controlled intervention trials and observational studies show that cutting back moderately on sodium helps lower blood pressure. The catch is that some individuals have a much greater blood pressure response to salt than others. About half those with high blood pressure are "salt sensitive." But only 10 percent of the total American population falls into this category. As yet, we can't predict if you're salt sensitive until you develop high blood pressure and reduce your intake. Since there is no harm in moderately cutting back on dietary sodium, this is widely recommended. There's also a theory that a high level of sodium over time is what causes rising blood pressure as the body ages. So if your blood pressure is normal now, cutting back to a reasonable amount of sodium may help keep it that way.

The Great Sodium Debate

Figuring out what a "reasonable" amount of sodium is has turned out to be a major public health debate. Many public and private organizations say Americans should consume no more than 2,400 mg of sodium a day. That equals about 6 grams or 1½ teaspoons of salt (sodium chloride). The most recent U.S. Dietary Guidelines for Americans and the 1996 Dietary Guidelines for Healthy American Adults, from the American Heart Association, both suggest a limit of 2,400 mg.

Not too long ago 2,200 milligrams of sodium was considered a significant dietary restriction. Hospitalized patients were given individualized counseling from registered dietitians on how to follow such a plan before they could be discharged to go home. A more reasonable estimate of moderate sodium for healthy adults with normal blood pressure is probably in the range of 3,000 to 5,000 mg per day.

It's hard to eat less than 5,000 milligrams of sodium if you rely on processed convenience foods and/or often eat meals away from home. Take a look at the sodium content of McDonald's items below. Do you have high blood pressure? Are you at risk for high blood pressure because it runs in your family? If your answer is yes to either of these questions, it's worthwhile to consider ways to eat less sodium. However, if you have more pressing areas to work on—maintaining a healthy weight, changing your fat intake—don't make lowering sodium your primary focus.

Salt Sense

Salt is an acquired taste. The more you eat, the more you want. Savvy salt sleuths know that you can't tell the sodium content of a food by the way it tastes. Salt that is added to foods after cooking provides a huge amount of flavor. That's because the salt is placed right on your taste buds when it goes into your mouth. Salt or sodium-based seasonings that are cooked into food or added as preservatives don't have the same dramatic effect. The bottom line: If you need to add salt, do it at the table, not in cooking. Look at these shocking comparisons:

Where's the McSalt?

McDonald's Item	mg of Sodium	Fascinating Facts
French fries, regular size	135	Yes, these fries were salted after frying.
Milkshake, small chocolate or vanilla	250	The sodium in your shake is from added preservatives.
Hamburger, regular	580	The condiments—ketchup and pickle—supply most of the sodium here.
Quarter Pounder	820	More condiments and more bread mean more sodium.
Bacon, Egg, and Cheese Biscuit	1310	Yes, it's the highest-sodium item on the menu.

Source: Adapted from McDonald's Corporation, 1998

LINK UP to **http://www.nhlbi.nih.gov,** the National Heart, Lung, and Blood Institute site, for the latest information and research on blood pressure.

Why you need it: sodium regulates fluid balance and helps keep your blood pH normal, regulates blood pressure, helps send nerve impulses.

For optimal health: 5,000 mg or less of sodium (¼ teaspoon of salt contains 500 mg)

Best natural food sources: all foods contain some sodium

Fortified foods: most processed foods have moderate to high amounts of added sodium; highly processed foods can have extremely high amounts of added sodium

Minimum toxic dose: not known; varies by person and health status. May cause fluid retention; swelling; and for those individuals who are sodium sensitive, may raise blood pressure.

Selected Studies
- The Trials of Hypertension Prevention, Phase II (TOHP II) study, found that short-term sodium reduction and weight loss made a difference in improving blood pressure. Each change lowered blood pressure in those who were overweight and had slightly elevated blood pressure. However, the study group did not fully maintain their weight loss and sodium reduction over three to four years, and the effects on blood pressure reduction were lessened (*Annals of Epidemiology,* March 1995). It's long-term lifestyle changes that improve overall health and can reduce blood pressure and weight.

- The Dietary Approaches to Stop Hypertension (DASH) studied the effects on blood pressure of entire eating plans. DASH found that, without testing the effect of salt reduction, a diet lower in fat and higher in vegetables, fruits, and low-fat dairy foods significantly reduced blood pressure in those with normal to slightly elevated pressures (*Archives of Internal Medicine,* February 1999). Just one more huge study that proves eating lots of fruits and vegetables has definite health benefits.

- The most recently published study is the Trial of Nonpharmacologic Interventions in the Elderly (TONE). This multicenter clinical trial reported that lifestyle changes of dietary salt reduction, weight loss, or both together reduced blood pressure in older patients with hypertension. Most study participants were able to decrease the amount of medication they were taking to lower blood pressure (*American Journal of Cardiology,* December 1998). It's not only more healthful, but cheaper to lower blood pressure by eating nutritious foods than by taking medication.

TRACE ELEMENTS

Iron

Just as iron helps form the skeleton of a skyscraper, it help support your strength and vitality. Between 1992 and 1995 the idea that too much iron causes heart attacks was promoted. Iron was almost considered a toxic poison until worldwide population studies were completed that proved no link between iron and heart disease.

There is one genetic disease related to too much iron. The Centers for Disease Control (CDC) estimates that over 1.5 million Americans have heterozygous hemochromatosis. This recessive genetic defect causes absorption and storage of iron at levels well above normal. There are no obvious side effects until iron stores in the brain, heart, liver, and pancreases begin to cause organ failure. Early symptoms usually don't appear until the age of 30.

For many people, especially women, it's hard to get enough iron. It's almost impossible for pregnant or breast-feeding women to meet their increased iron requirements. That's one of the reasons why prenatal supplements are so important. Before birth, a baby has just nine months to store up enough iron to last until it's time to start solid foods. Breast milk is naturally low in iron. New moms also need to replace iron stores that were depleted during pregnancy and to make up for the additional blood lost during delivery and recovery from the birthing process. Women with heavy menstrual blood losses may need the same high levels of iron (30 mg/day) as pregnant women.

If you think you might be iron deficient, ask for a transferrin saturation or total iron binding capacity blood test. If those test results are out of the range of normal, then the more expensive serum ferritin test should be given. The serum ferritin test is the best way to measure how much iron is stored in your organs. All of these tests are more sensitive than the usual hemoglobin or hematocrit.

Iron is found in both animal and plant foods. There's no dispute that heme sources of iron in meat are much better absorbed than nonheme plant iron. However, if you eat a food high in vitamin C with a plant food that contains iron, you can dramatically increase absorption of this mineral. For example, add some orange sections to your spinach salad or mix red or green peppers into your favorite bean dish. Lug out your old cast-iron cooking skillets. Cast-iron pots and pans add a small but significant amount of iron to the foods cooked in them. Yes, some iron (a 2 to 4 percent total increase) from the pan is deposited into your food during cooking.

Why you need it: iron carries oxygen throughout the body in both blood and muscle tissue.

For optimal health: 10 to 30 mg/day of iron. Lower levels are for children, men, and postmenopausal women. Higher levels are for women with heavy periods or those who are pregnant or breast-feeding.

Best natural food sources: beef, clams, oysters, and soybeans (cooked)

Fortified foods: bread, pasta, white rice, ready-to-eat cereals, farina, and oatmeal

Minimum toxic dose: 30 mg/day of iron or more may cause constipation, stomach upset, abdominal pain, or bloody diarrhea. In children, toxic doses can be severe enough to cause convulsions, coma, or death.

Selected Studies
Researchers at the National Council for Health Statistics analyzed data from the most recent Nutrition and Health Examination Survey that studied what more than 25,000 people ate. They found iron deficiency in 9 percent of toddlers, 9 to 11 percent of teenage girls and women of childbearing age, and 7 percent of women older than 70. That translates into 700,000 toddlers and 7.8 million women (*Journal of the American Medical Association,* March 1997). If you are in one of the high-risk groups for low iron intake, have your blood tested at your next doctor visit.

Chromium
The mineral chromium is the same stuff that makes old-fashioned car bumpers shiny. It also helps you shine when you need to work or play hard. Because it helps regulate insulin, chromium is important in helping you maintain peak energy under pressure. That doesn't mean it will make you stronger, smarter, or capable of more than is normal for you.

Borderline chromium deficiency is thought to be common, especially in older people. There seems to be a connection between chromium deficiency and the high rates of diabetes as you age. It might be linked to the fact that diets high in simple sugars tend to increase chromium losses. But that doesn't mean that high-sugar diets cause diabetes. Almost all adult-onset diabetes is caused by weight gain. Getting adequate amounts of chromium may decrease insulin injection doses and improve how certain diabetics handle glucose. If you want to know more about chromium picolinate or alternative supplements, see Chapter 7 for details.

Why you need it: chromium works with insulin to help your body use glucose and maintain normal blood sugar levels.

For optimal health: 50 to 200 mcg/day of chromium

Best natural food sources: brewer's yeast, corn on the cob, beef, apples, sweet potato, eggs, and prunes

Fortified foods: none

Minimum toxic dose: none known from dietary sources. Long-term environmental exposure from electroplating, steel manufacturing, cement manufacturing, glass and jewelry making, photography, textile dyeing, and wood preserving may cause skin problems, liver and kidney damage, or cancer.

Selected Studies

Widespread chromium deficiency in the general population was determined to be the result of two factors. First, most people don't eat many food sources of chromium and second, the more sugar you eat, the more chromium you lose (*Progress in Clinical and Biological Research,* vol. 380, 1993). If your diet is high in sugar, be sure to include lots of chromium-rich foods and include chromium in your multivitamin-mineral supplement.

Copper

If your water pipes are made of copper, you're in luck—drinking water that runs through copper pipes may add a significant amount of this hard-to-get mineral to your intake. Copper's main priority is to aid breathing. It works to help regulate the absorption and release of iron. Copper and iron are good buddies; they rely on each other being there to work efficiently.

Why you need it: copper helps form hemoglobin; keeps bones, blood vessels, and nerves healthy.

For optimal health: 2 to 3 mg/day of copper

Best natural food sources: barley, crab, lobster, and oysters

Fortified foods: none

Minimum toxic dose: 20 mg/day of copper or more may cause anemia, muscle aches, nausea, vomiting, liver damage, or coma. Wilson's disease, an inherited disorder, causes excess copper accumulation in body tissues. Treatment requires a low-copper diet and medication to bind copper before it can be absorbed.

Selected Studies

Researchers studying animal models and cell cultures have found a link between copper deficiency and a reduction in immunity. They found that even a marginal copper deficiency can have a negative impact (*American Journal of Clinical Nutrition,* May 1998). This is not a human study, but it suggests new information about copper status that might be valuable for assessing nutrient and immunity status in humans. Remember that taking too much zinc can cause a copper deficiency.

Fluoride

Do you have a mouthful of gleaming silver fillings proving you grew up without benefit of fluoridated water? For over sixty years, the dental benefits of fluoride have been known. If you drank fluoridated water as a child, you have 50 to 70 percent fewer cavities than your peers who didn't have fluoride. Yet there are still naysayers who think fluoridated water is the cause of many cancers.

The biggest source of fluoride is usually the local water supply. Half of all U.S. water supplies are fluoridated. Those that aren't are homes that rely on well water or nonmunicipal water sources. Most bottled water does not contain fluoride. Low doses of fluoride are beneficial to the dental health of adults as well as children. If you don't know if your water is fluoridated, call your local water department to find out. A typical amount added is 0.7 to 1.2 mg per liter of water. The American Academy of Pediatrics recommends that all breast-fed infants and babies using reconstituted formula in households where the water is not fluoridated start supplements at 6 months.

Many experts recommend continuing with supplements until age 16, especially if you drink and cook exclusively with unfluoridated tap or bottled water. Unlike most nutrient supplements, fluoride is available only by prescription from your doctor or dentist.

Why you need it: fluoride hardens tooth enamel and protects teeth from decay; strengthens bone.

For optimal health: 1.5 to 4 mg/day of fluoride

Best natural food sources: not widely found in foods and varies with soil content where foods are grown

Fortified foods: municipal drinking water (check with your local water supplier)

Minimum toxic dose: 10 mg/day of fluoride or more may cause stomach cramps, vomiting, diarrhea, tremors. Long-term high doses cause mottled teeth, brittle bones, and increased frequency of broken bones. Toothpaste with fluoride should be spit out and not swallowed; only use a pea-size amount for children.

Iodine

Iodine is known as a micronutrient, for good reason. The average person needs only a teaspoon of it over the course of an entire lifetime. But if you don't get even that small amount, it can cause big trouble. "Lack of iodine is the world's leading cause of preventable mental retardation and can cause population-wide drops in IQ in areas where deficiency is common," according to Dr. Glen Maberly of the Rollins School of Public Health at Emory University.

"When it rains, it pours" is the Morton Salt motto. With the case of iodine, it's ironically true. Iodized salt is the most recognizable source of iodine, a nutrient once scarce in many parts of the country. Adding iodine to table salt began in 1924 in Michigan to help prevent the spread of goiter that was common in the Great Lakes region. The practice soon spread across the United States.

In the 1970s, physicians began to notice that when they used radioactive iodine for diagnostic testing, the thyroid gland absorbed less than the expected amount of this marker. That's because the dramatic increase of iodine in the food supply resulted in most people being saturated with all the iodine their bodies could hold. In the 1974 total diet study completed by the FDA, the range of iodine intakes for adults was estimated at 500 to 800 mg/day—more than four to five and a half times the recommended amount. Rates for infants and toddlers were six to thirteen times the RDA. Those estimates were based on the assumption that noniodized salt was used in cooking and at the table. Use of iodized salt would add another 300 mg of iodine daily.

Where is all the added iodine coming from? You might be surprised:

- A Big Mac Value Meal has almost three times the adult RDA for iodine.
- A frozen fried chicken dinner can have between six and twenty-nine times the recommended intake.
- Multivitamin supplements that use red food color #3 (which is more than 50 percent iodine) have 100 to 150 more milligrams of iodine than is noted on the label. That's because when an ingredient in a product is included as an additive (a coloring agent in this example), the manufacturer doesn't need to include any nutrients it might contribute. (No, it doesn't make sense.) Since two other red dyes have been banned, the use of red food color #3 has increased more than 50 percent.
- Dairy foods contribute almost 40 percent of all the iodine we eat. Cow teats, farm machinery, and processing equipment are all sanitized and cleaned with iodine-containing chemicals.
- Food processors often use iodine-based chemicals for cleaning and sanitizing. According to the FDA, significant amounts of iodine end up in foods like grains, cereals, sugars, jellies, and puddings.

This overconsumption of iodine has been blamed for the declining success in treating people with hyperthyroidism. Treatment today is only 17 percent effective, compared to 60 percent successful treatment with antithyroid medications a generation ago. People with Hashimoto's thyroiditis can have their thyroid function blocked if they get too much iodine. Iodine-containing asthma medications used by mothers during pregnancy have caused goiters in newborns.

But wait! A 1988 to 1994 sample of almost 34,000 Americans released in October of 1998 found that 12 percent of Americans had low levels of iodine in their urine (a laboratory indicator of iodine intake), says the CDC. In 1974, only 3 percent of the U.S. population had low urine iodine concentrations. But 1974 was the same year the FDA's data said we were all getting way too much.

The message is if you eat a lot of processed foods, you might be better off with plain salt. If you avoid processed foods and are frugal with the salt shaker, choose iodized salt from the grocery shelf.

Why you need it: iodine helps your body form thyroid hormones, which are vital to physical growth and development. Thyroid hormones control metabolism; improve mental functioning; and give you healthier hair, skin, nails, and teeth.

For optimal health: 150 mcg/day of iodine

Best natural food sources: not widely found in foods and varies with soil content where foods are grown. Saltwater fish and seafood provide modest amounts of iodine.

Fortified foods: iodized table salt; food processors use iodized salt and sanitizing solutions that contribute iodine indirectly to foods

Minimum toxic dose: 2 mg/day of iodine or more may cause irregular heartbeat, confusion, goiter (swollen neck or throat), and bloody or tarry stools

Selenium

In 1979, researchers first described an association between selenium deficiency and heart-muscle disease. Often called cardiomyopathy, selenium deficiency causes enlargement of the heart and heart failure. It primarily affects women in their childbearing years and children.

It's interesting to note that a selenium deficiency during pregnancy can have irreversible effects on your baby's development and growth. The most dramatic consequence of selenium deficiency during fetal growth is damage to the immune system.

Why you need it: selenium works as an antioxidant with vitamin E.

For optimal health: 200 mcg/day of selenium

Best natural food sources: salmon and haddock. Accurate levels of selenium in cultivated foods are not available as selenium content varies with the soil levels of this mineral.

Fortified foods: none

Minimum toxic dose: 700 mcg/day of selenium or more from inorganic sodium selenite may cause hair loss, fingernail loss, fatigue, nausea, or nerve damage.

Manganese

Manganese isn't a glamorous nutrient, but it is shrouded in mystery. We don't know much about manganese because few scientists are interested in studying it. The first reported deficiency of manganese was not noted until 1972.

Why you need it: manganese is a vital part of many enzymes; promotes normal growth and development.

For optimal health: 2.5 to 5.0 mg/day of manganese

Best natural food sources: whole grains, pineapple, strawberries, lentils, kale, tea

Fortified foods: none

Minimum toxic dose: not known, but large doses may cause depression, delusions, hallucinations, impotence, or insomnia and may interfere with iron absorption

Selected Studies
A University of Wisconsin study of forty-seven women eating typical American diets found that those who ate more plant-based iron (nonheme) instead of heme iron, found in meat, had lower manganese blood levels. Foods that contain lots of manganese-like leafy green vegetables, whole-grain bread, and cereals, also often contain large amounts of nonheme iron (*American Journal of Clinical Nutrition*, November 1992). Women who eat very little meat may have low blood levels of manganese that cannot be raised by eating additional plant sources of manganese.

Molybdenum

If you haven't heard of molybdenum, don't worry. It's the least known of all essential minerals. It's also among one of the scarcest minerals found in the earth's crust.

Why you need it: molybdenum promotes normal growth and development, aids in enzyme conversion of uric acid, and helps iron metabolism.

For optimal health: 75 to 250 mcg/day of molybdenum

Best natural food sources: leafy dark green vegetables, legumes, and milk

Fortified foods: breads and cold cereals

Minimum toxic dose: 1 mg/day of molybdenum or more may cause excessive loss of copper in urine; 10 to 15 mg per day may cause gout-like symptoms.

Zinc

Your body has about the same amount of zinc as a 4-inch galvanized nail (1.5 to 2.5 gm). Unlike other trace minerals, zinc is not stored in the body but acts as a functioning nutrient. Zinc is a party animal—it likes to circulate and doesn't take time to rest.

Zinc helps put zip into your immune system. Even a mild zinc deficiency can increase your risk of infection. Stomach acid is important for zinc efficiency. Medications or health problems that decrease available stomach acid may limit absorption of zinc. If you have children who like to put coins in their mouths, beware of newer U.S. pennies. The zinc now added to pennies poses a new risk for stomach ulcers if a child (or anyone) swallows them.

Getting the right amount of zinc is similar to walking a tightrope. It's a fine line between too much and not enough—with hazards for any missteps. Loading up with zinc for more than a week can weaken your immune system, lower your HDL (good) cholesterol, and trigger a copper deficiency. Tumor cells demand zinc for growth, and when the supply is plentiful they thrive. If you have cancer, zinc supplements are usually not recommended. Pesky skin conditions, including dandruff flaking and psoriasis, speed up zinc losses. Since zinc is such a circulator, you lose it when your skin rubs off or you comb out that "flaky white stuff." If you substantially increase your calcium intake, you may need more zinc. Vegetarians sometimes have a hard time getting enough zinc. That's because soy foods and whole grains are high in substances that are natural inhibitors of zinc absorption. Zinc found in animal foods, especially red meat, seafood, and eggs, is absorbed up to four times more effectively than zinc found in plant foods.

Why you need it: zinc forms protein in the body; helps wound healing, blood formation, and general growth and maintenance of all tissues. It is part of many enzymes and is essential for most metabolic processes. Zinc also maintains normal taste and smell sensations.

For optimal health: 15 to 20 mg/day of zinc, people who take extra calcium supplements need the higher levels. Don't take extra zinc without a doctor's supervision.

Best natural food sources: beef, lamb, oysters, pork, and veal

Fortified foods: most fortified ready-to-eat cereals, hot and cold, contain about 10 percent of the RDA.

Minimum toxic dose: 30 mg/day of zinc or more may cause drowsiness, nausea, vomiting, diarrhea, impaired coordination, or restlessness; weaken the immune system; lower HDL (good) cholesterol; decrease copper and iron levels.

Selected Studies

At the Cleveland Clinic, 100 people who had developed colds in the last twenty-four hours were told to suck on zinc gluconate–glycine lozenges every two hours. Half the study group took real zinc lozenges, the other half were given placebo lozenges. Those who took the zinc lozenges had colds that lasted 4.4 days compared to 7.6 days for the placebo-takers (*Journal of the American Medical Association,* June 1998). If you don't mind the taste, zinc lozenges may help shorten your cold. However, in November 1999, the Federal Trade Commission successfully settled a suit against the home shopping network QVC and the makers of Cold-Eeze, Cold Eezer, and Kids-Eeze Bubble-Gum because their ads said severity of symptoms are reduced. They are not.

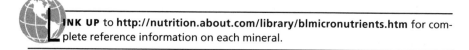

LINK UP to http://nutrition.about.com/library/blmicronutrients.htm for complete reference information on each mineral.

Dueling Minerals

If you take too much of one vitamin or mineral, it can decrease your ability to absorb other nutrients. Here are some of the most common interactions:

If you take too much:	You might become deficient in:
Calcium	Magnesium, Iron, and Zinc
Copper	Zinc
Iron	Phosphorus and Zinc
Manganese	Iron
Molybdenum	Copper and Zinc
Phosphorus	Calcium
Zinc	Copper

Mineral Needs for Special Situations

Nutrient	Highest Federal Standard (RDA or DV)	Optimal Intake	Individuals with Special Needs*
Calcium	1,000–1,200 mg	1,000–1,500 mg	Milk avoiders, those on very low-calorie diets, and people over 55—especially postmenopausal women
Phosphorus	700–1,200 mg	800–1,200 mg	People with kidney disease or problems of the digestive tract
Magnesium	310–420 mg	350–500 mg	People over 70, very active individuals, diabetics, and those on very low-calorie diets
Iron	15 mg	10–30 mg	Women with heavy menstrual blood losses and those on very low-calorie diets
Zinc	15 mg	15–25 mg	People over 70, some vegetarians, very active adults, and diabetics
Iodine	150 mcg	Not known	Not known
Copper	1.5–3 mg	2–3 mg	Premature babies and people who take large amounts of vitamin C or zinc from supplements
Manganese	2–5 mg	Not known	Those on very low-calorie diets
Fluoride	3.2–3.8 mg	2–4 mg	People who don't have fluoridated water, especially children 6 months to 16 years old
Chromium	50–200 mcg	50–200 mg	Those over 70 and people on very low-calorie diets
Molybdenum	75–250 mcg	Not known	Not known
Selenium	70 mcg	100–200 mg	Women in their childbearing years and children

*Note: Pregnant and breast-feeding women, alcoholics, and drug abusers have increased needs for most nutrients.

SUPPLEMENT SCENARIOS

There are a variety of ways to optimize your intake of important nutrients.

1. Don't supplement. Eat a wide variety of fruits, vegetables, and grains every day. Choose skim or low-fat milk and dairy products for adequate calcium. Eat lean red meat and seafood at least several times a week for their high mineral contents.

2. Take vitamin E and/or calcium supplements daily. It's almost impossible to get optimal amounts of vitamin E from foods. If you can't or won't drink milk or eat other calcium-rich foods, a calcium supplement is worth considering.

3. Take a multivitamin and mineral supplement daily. If you are making smart food choices, the extra amounts in a multivitamin will push you toward the optimal amounts of most nutrients.

4. Take a multivitamin and mineral supplement, along with vitamin E and calcium, if you need them.

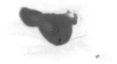

7
Alternative Supplements

Many alternative supplements are drugs—they're just regulated differently. Because a product has been popular and on the market for years doesn't mean it's safe or effective. How much do you really know about the supplements you take? People usually spend more time researching their next car or computer purchase than selecting their supplements.

Don't be afraid to call a manufacturer's toll-free number and ask questions. The National Council for Responsible Health Information (formerly the National Council Against Health Fraud) investigated performance-enhancing claims made by supplement companies. Here's what they found:

- Misrepresentation: often manufacturers use information that is not 100 percent accurate. Advertising and public relations firms frequently determine what claims and slogans to use.
- Research currently under way: when asked for research data, many companies say they are in the process of conducting research. If they can't or won't give specific details or put you in touch with researchers, be wary.
- Not for public review: when you are denied access to documentation for label and marketing claims, it's likely they don't have any.
- Testimonials: everybody loves a good story. Celebrities, sports personalities, and even politicians have been used in this popular sales technique. Testimonials are usually paid endorsements.
- Patent or patent pending: the manufacturer thinks the product is unique or special. It may be. That doesn't mean it is effective or safe.
- Inappropriately referenced material: a lengthy list of research studies looks impressive. Often studies cited are poorly designed, don't prove anything, have never been published or reviewed, don't relate to the topic, or may not even exist.

All the products in this chapter have one thing in common: They are relatively new supplements. They don't have the history of herbal products or the wealth of investigation and research supporting many of the vitamins and minerals. This doesn't make them bad; we just know less about how they may or may not act to improve or impair health.

AMINO ACIDS

Regardless of what the supplement ads say, extra protein or amino acids will not increase your muscle mass or improve athletic performance. Because amino acids compete with each other for absorption, too much of one can decrease absorption and utilization of the others. In 1974 amino acid supplements were removed from the Food and Drug Administration's GRAS (Generally Recognized As Safe) list. Currently the only approved use for amino acids is as part of medical foods such as intravenous feedings for people who need special formulas because of health problems like kidney or liver disease.

Most amino acid supplements are made from egg protein or animal protein. They can be readily purchased as capsules, tablets, and powders. Small amounts of protein foods like milk, meat, or eggs can supply significantly more amino acids at a fraction of the cost of supplements.

Selected Studies
Research on U.S. Marine officer candidates showed that marines who were given amino acid supplements performed exactly the same—before, during, and after the study—as those who were given a placebo (*Medicine and Science in Sports,* April 1996). If it doesn't work for "America's best," it won't work for you.

Arginine

This amino acid has been proclaimed by its promoters as "being able to cause weight loss overnight." The stimulation of growth hormone is the supposed action that causes you to shed pounds while you dream of getting thin on arginine (ARE-gin-een). While it's true that arginine can stimulate the secretion of growth hormone, it must be taken in massive amounts—more than can be found in commercial supplements. But growth hormone doesn't have anything to do with weight loss. As far back as 1978 arginine (along with cystine, treonine, tyrosine, leucine, methionine, phenylalanine, and valine to name just a few) was investigated by a scientific panel and was found to be worthless as a weight loss aid.

Selected Studies
A Mayo Clinic study found that the dietary supplement L-arginine improves chest pain symptoms in patients with early heart disease. People who took an L-arginine pill every day for six months had significantly less chest pain and

improved coronary blood flow than those who took a placebo. Investigators studied twenty-six participants without significant heart disease and reported that improvements began after one week of use and continued for the six-month study (*Circulation,* July 1999). It's thought that L-arginine, through a series of chemical reactions, acts on the lining of blood vessels to relax the vessel wall and may inhibit the buildup of platelets and plaques.

L-tryptophan

L-tryptophan (el-TRIP-toe-fan) is perhaps the most infamous of all supplements. Pills containing this amino acid were marketed as a solution for people with insomnia. More than 1,200 individuals who took tryptophan developed a painful connective tissue and blood disease called eosinophilia-myalgia syndrome. At least thirty-eight people died from exposure to a contaminant in the supplement. A variant of tryptophan is now sold as 5-HTP and may also be contaminated with an impurity known as "peak X." Contamination of supplements is common, says Roseanne Philen, an epidemiologist with the Centers for Disease Control. Some supplements have contaminants added deliberately. Herbal remedies may be laced with real drugs to give them an extra punch. For example, arthritis products spiked with painkillers, tranquilizers, or steroids have been discovered.

PABA

What's sunscreen doing in my supplement? Para amino benzoic acid (PABA) is best known for its work as a sunscreen. It helps block out skin-damaging ultraviolet rays. It's also an ingredient used by your body to make the vitamin folic acid. Oral PABA supplements won't help you make more folic acid though; only plants and certain bacteria can do that. PABA supplements also won't make you sun-safe from the inside out. If you do take PABA supplements and sulfa antibiotics at the same time, PABA can cancel the antibiotic's effectiveness.

SAM-e

SAM-e (S-adenosyl-methionine) is one of the newest supplements to be stocked on store shelves and claims to help sufferers of osteoarthritis and depression. This compound is produced by your body from the amino acid methionine. With help from vitamin B12 and folic acid, SAM-e helps with the maintenance of cell membranes, removal of toxic substances from the body, and the production of mood-enhancing neurotransmitters such as noradrenaline, serotonin, and possibly dopamine, according to recent marketing claims.

SAM-e has been used for two decades in Europe to treat osteoarthritis and depression. It first was discovered in the 1950s at the National Institutes of Health. In the 1970s, an Italian lab learned to produce it in cell cultures, and studied its use as an antidepressant. Some of the first patients who were given SAM-e for depression also suffered with osteoarthritis. The anti-arthritic potential of SAM-e was realized when some people reported relief from their joint pain as well as their depression. SAM-e may work by rebuilding worn-down joint cartilage through increasing production of a substance called proteoglycans. SAM-e has few, if any, known side effects. It only takes four to ten days to provide relief compared to several weeks required for prescription antidepressants or St. John's wort.

However, there are no current plans to conduct double-blind, placebo-controlled studies, which are necessary in the United States to prove the effectiveness of medicines. As with many U.S. dietary supplements, its main appeal is as an alternative to drugs. In Europe, SAM-e is sold *only* as a prescription drug. In the United States, it's being marketed as a dietary supplement with claims that it promotes "joint health" and "emotional well-being." A month's supply (400 mg/day) can cost between $75 and $90. If you have moderate or severe depression, self-medication with SAM-e is not recommended.

ENZYMES

Enzymes are proteins that act like biological spark plugs for chemical reactions in your body. You make more than enough of your own enzymes. In fact, a single cell contains thousands of enzymes, each with a specific job. Taking enzymes in supplement form is useless because enzymes are almost all broken down into their amino acid building blocks during digestion. Enzymes can't provide any biologic benefit when they are broken down. Certain digestive enzymes, like lactase, may be taken orally if you are deficient in that particular enzyme (e.g., lactose intolerant). Digestive enzymes are the only ones that can work and survive in the digestive tract and be used effectively. People with chronic pancreas disease may need to take supplemental digestive enzymes. That's because the pancreas is where these enzymes are manufactured. Because they are protein molecules, enzymes are inactivated by heat, often at temperatures as low as 115 to 120°F.

CoQ-10

Ubiquone, or CoQ-10, is found in every cell of every plant and animal on earth. Each of your cells contains a miniature power factory called the mitochondrion. This is where the energy your body needs is made. CoQ-10 helps regulate the electrical currents that fuel this factory. Imagine a string of holiday lights. If one of the bulbs doesn't work, the others go out, too. It's CoQ-10's job to get in there and replace any defective or empty sockets to keep the system functioning.

There are many stories about how CoQ-10 can enhance athletic performance or decrease fatigue. A few athletes and coaches firmly believe that CoQ-10 supplementation benefits performance, and the result has been a virtual marketing blitz. However, credible scientific evidence to support these claims is lacking. Studies have shown that supplementation with CoQ-10 is beneficial for some people with heart failure. Research on healthy athletes, however, doesn't show any improvement in performance with CoQ-10 supplementation.

Selected Studies

Eighteen highly trained male triathletes and cyclists took daily doses of either a supplement capsule or a placebo for four weeks and then exercised to exhaustion. The supplement contained 100 mg CoQ-10, 500 mg cytochrome C, 100 mg inosine, and 200 IU vitamin E. After four weeks of no supplements, they started another four weeks of supplement or placebo—opposite of what they had before—and tested again. The test was ninety minutes of running on a treadmill, followed by cycling on a stationary bike until exhaustion set in. No significant differences in stamina between the groups were found (*International Journal of Sport Nutrition,* September 1997). CoQ-10 does not seem to have any effect on athletic performance.

ERGOGENIC AIDS

The quest for more energy, bigger muscles, and less body fat is a popular one. Ergogenic (err-go-JEN-ick) aids sometimes help fuel this search. Ergogenic aids are broadly defined as techniques or substances used for enhancing athletic performance. Ergogenic aids include food, supplements, drugs, training methods, or psychological manipulation. They range from use of reasonable techniques such as carbohydrate loading to illegal and unsafe approaches like anabolic-androgenic steroid use.

Protein is the most popular and enduring ergogenic aid. The notion that massive amounts of protein are necessary during training has evolved from ancient beliefs that great strength could be obtained by eating the raw meat of lions, tigers, or other animals that displayed great fighting strength. Although few athletes consume raw meat today, the idea that "you are what you eat" is still widely promoted by food faddists. The problem is that some athletes go too far with ergogenic aids.

SPORT FUEL: NECESSARY OR NOT?

The explosive sports food market beckons elite athletes and everyday exercisers alike. But are these high-tech fuels really necessary for the average person? Probably not, say sports medicine experts. What most athletes need is calories and water, plain and simple. ▶

Sports Beverages

Hype: Touted as the ideal replacement for water loss during exercise.

Help: You can replace lost fluids with any liquid, but water is best unless you need or want extra calories. Eating any regular foods after exercise can replace lost sodium and stimulate thirst.

Harm: Constant consumption of sports drinks or any other beverage high in sugar can promote tooth decay if you don't brush your teeth frequently.

Energy Bars

Hype: Advertised as instant energizers.

Help: The bars are convenient to carry, but many are only reduced-fat candy bars with some added nutrients.

Harm: None really, except that some bars have close to 500 calories. Be sure to drink plenty of water to help improve nutrient absorption. However, some energy bars how contain herbs that could cause adverse reactions in sensitive individuals.

Protein Powders

Hype: Protein and amino acid supplements claim to enhance muscle development.

Help: None. Only physical training builds muscle.

Harm: Too much protein can be harmful and may stress your kidneys and lead to dehydration. Taking individual amino acids can also cause nutrient imbalances. Some protein powders contain added herbs and megadoses of vitamins and minerals.

Goos and Gels

Hype: Quick energy (calories) for endurance athletes.

Help: The tubes and packets that hold these products are convenient for long-distance runners and cyclists. Most are nutritionally equivalent to jelly or jam.

Harm: High-priced source of calories. Be sure to drink plenty of fluid when using goos or gels or you could develop cramps.

Glycerol

Hype: A way to "hyperhydrate" or store large amounts of water before training or competition.

Help: Glycerol, usually found in fatty foods, chemically attracts and holds water like a sponge.

Harm: May cause bloating and feelings of nausea. While glycerol does enhance fluid retention, there is no proof that this has a positive effect on athletic performance.

Chromium Picolinate

Need to slim down and bulk up at the same time? Patented, pricey, designer-labeled chromium picolinate (pick-OH-lin-ate) isn't a better choice than ordinary chromium that's found in food and many multivitamin and mineral supplements. It's true that picolinate is a compound that, when combined with a metal like chromium, enhances the ability of that mineral to get into the body's cells. Chromium picolinate is remarkably stable in the body, which may explain why it is more readily absorbed than chromium obtained through regular dietary sources. But this stability may also allow it to be accumulated in cells in its DNA-damaging form.

Probably what piques interest in chromium picolinate is the lure of losing fat and gaining muscle tone without any effort. But the studies these claims are loosely based on used crude measures of testing body fat that were not reliable and have not been duplicated by other research. When the USDA Human Nutrition Research Center tried to replicate the data using sophisticated, state-of-the-art techniques to measure body composition, there was no difference between those who took chromium picolinate for two months and those who did not.

Chromium picolinate does help insulin transfer glucose and other nutrients from the bloodstream to cells. If the glucose doesn't move readily into your cells after eating, it keeps your blood sugar unnecessarily high and can result in diabetes. But any modest reduction caused by chromium picolinate in your blood sugar level isn't enough to bring it back to the normal range.

Selected Studies

Dr. John Vincent, a University of Alabama researcher, reported at the American Chemical Society's annual meeting in March 1999 that the popular dietary supplement chromium picolinate may damage DNA, possibly increasing the risk of cancer. Vincent looked at the chemical reaction among vitamin C, other compounds, and chromium picolinate at 100 times less than the concentration found in human body tissue after long-term use. The researchers found that the reaction produces chromium II, which interacts with oxygen to produce hydroxyl radicals, agents known to cause mutations and other types of DNA damage. Careful investigation into the effects of long-term diet supplementation with chromium picolinate is needed. Chromium picolinate supplements that are combined with vitamin C supplements may be the most dangerous.

The Creatine Craze

It's not unusual for high school and college coaches to see several student athletes before practice huddled together measuring out a small amount of a white powdery substance. No, it's not cocaine, it's the other c-word: creatine. Baseball batting demons Mark McGwire and Sammy Sosa helped fuel the creatine craze toward the end of the 1998 slug-fest season when they both admitted using this performance-enhancing potion.

Creatine is found naturally in animal muscle tissue and is named after the Greek word for flesh. Creatine monohydrate is taken up by muscle cells and converted to creatine phosphate, where it is stored until it's needed to make chemical energy. If plenty of creatine isn't available from the foods you eat, it is easily made by the liver and kidneys from a few amino acids (arginine, glycine, and methionine).

When certain athletes supplement with extra amounts of creatine, their muscles can produce more quick energy—but only in highly explosive activities or those with quick repetitive movements. If you need to bat a ball, lift heavy weights, or tackle your opponent to the ground, you might gain a competitive edge with creatine. If you're an endurance athlete such as a distance runner, swimmer, or triathlete, creatine won't help. Use of creatine by nonathletes is senseless.

According to sports nutrition expert Dr. Chris Rosenbloom, a professor at the University of Georgia, creatine supplementation:

- appears to benefit athletes during high-intensity, intermittent exercise. Improvements are most noticeable in athletes who have low creatine stores (i.e., vegetarian athletes or those who eat little meat).
- may enhance training sessions, allowing athletes to train at higher intensity.
- is associated with an increase in body mass, with the average weight gain of two to six pounds in as little as a week. It is unclear if the added weight is from extra water held in the muscles or from an increase in muscle mass. Most female athletes avoid this supplement like the plague. Extra pounds are a negative, undesirable side effect for many female athletes, especially those involved in endurance sports.

Most athletes take 20 to 25 grams a day during a weeklong "loading phase," in divided doses of 5 grams taken four or five times a day with food or a carbohydrate-containing beverage. The dose is tapered to 2 to 10 grams daily during the "maintenance phase." Extra water when supplementing with creatine is essential to prevent dehydration. Caffeine may diminish the ergogenic effect of creatine supplementation. Despite this, some of the commonly available powdered drink supplements contain both creatine and caffeine.

Claims of creatine's power have escalated beyond the science to support them. Athletes from a wide variety of sports are loading up with this expensive supplement. No long-term safety studies have been done, and most research is limited to just a few weeks of observation of creatine's effects on the body. That's unfortunate because more young athletes are taking creatine for longer periods of time. Reports in sports magazines and newspapers suggest as many as 25 percent of Major League Baseball players and up to 50 percent of National Football League players have tried creatine. Sales over the $200 million mark were reported for 1998.

Some creatine users report increased muscle cramping (especially during exercise in high heat), nausea, and other gastrointestinal disturbances. Creatine supplementation, in the dosages commonly used, results in urine concentrations that are ninety times greater than normal. Since creatine is filtered by the kidneys, there is the potential for significant kidney damage or disease with long-term use.

The bottom line is that no one can confidently state that prolonged creatine supplementation is safe. Use of creatine should be avoided, especially by young athletes, until more is known.

Selected Studies

Results from a small crossover random test showed that after a week of supplementing with creatine monohydrate, muscular performance was increased in athletes during high-intensity resistance exercise (*Journal of the American Dietetic Association,* July 1997). This study lasted only one week and didn't test for long-term side effects. Also, the results an average person may expect are significantly less than trained athletes.

LINK UP to http://www.ncaa.org/sports_sciences/drugtesting/banned_list.html for a list of all substances banned or restricted for athletes competing under the National Collegiate Athletic Association (NCAA) guidelines.

HORMONES

Hormones regulate overall body conditions, such as your blood sugar level (insulin hormone) and your metabolic rate (thyroid hormone). Hormones are chemical messengers that target specific tissues or organs. Unlike enzymes, not all hormones are made from protein, and they don't start chemical reactions, they just pass messages along. Hormones are highly potent chemical change agents and should not be taken without the recommendation of a health care provider. They are safest when purchased by prescription to ensure purity and quality.

DHEA

If you want something to slow aging, burn fat, build muscle, strengthen your immune system, ward off heart disease, prevent cancer, treat diabetes, delay Alzheimer's, or invigorate your sex life, dehydroepiandrosterone (dee-HI-drow-ep-EE-an-DOS-tur-own), or DHEA, is *not* the answer.

The FDA banned over-the-counter sales of DHEA in 1985 because of its potentially harmful side effects. Since then, it's reappeared in exactly the same form, as a "dietary supplement," which, of course, doesn't require FDA approval.

When you wake each day, the adrenal glands nestled on top of your kidneys release a form of DHEA into your bloodstream. As it merges into body tissue, DHEA is converted into tiny amounts of the sex hormones testosterone and estrogen. Normal DHEA levels in your body increase sharply at puberty, peak during early adulthood, and then gradually diminish with age until there's practically none left. So doesn't it make sense to add some back to recapture lost youth and vigor?

If you swallow these assumptions, you are risking your health. Not one of the above claims has been proven true in humans. However, there is plenty of evidence about the damage DHEA can cause. It has been shown to stimulate the enlargement of the prostate gland and to promote prostate cancer in men. In women, high levels of supplemental DHEA are linked to menstrual irregularities, masculinization (facial and body hair growth, deeper voices), and a higher risk of endometrial cancer. If you already have prostate or endometrial cancer, DHEA supplements can make it spread faster.

The bottom line: human hormones are powerful chemicals. Do-it-yourself DHEA hormone therapy is just plain D-U-M-B.

Melatonin Mania

Can't sleep? Have to work the night shift this week? Want a "natural" remedy for jet lag? Melatonin is a naturally occurring hormone that helps regulate sleep. Cued by nightfall, melatonin production begins at dusk and halts each morning as the sun rises. Your pineal gland (found in the brain) is the master controller of this rhythmic hormone that sets your sleeping and waking schedule. If you happen to live in a northern latitude where winter darkness extends beyond your normal wake-up time, you know melatonin's strong grip. Your body correctly senses it's still nighttime when it's dark outside and lures you to stay in bed.

Travelers may be able to decrease jet lag by taking melatonin at strategic times over a period of days and setting the body clock to a new time zone. Research seems to suggest that melatonin may decrease, but not eliminate, jet lag symptoms. Improvements such as decreased sleepiness and less morning tiredness may result.

There are preliminary data suggesting that low-dose melatonin supplements, given at specific times of day, can aid in the treatment of wintertime depression. However, the studies to date are too small and short-term to draw any conclusions.

OTHER COMMON ALTERNATIVES

A lot of strange and unusual things are eaten in the quest for health. Here are some common alternative supplements and what they will and won't do for you.

Bee Pollen

Bees keep busy bringing nectar and pollen to the hive—it's their full-time, lifelong job. They collect the pollen on body hairs, place it in "pollen baskets" on their legs, and then carry it back to the hive to be deposited in the honey cells. Pollen is essential for bees, but what about you? Proponents of bee pollen suggest that it can treat ailments ranging from allergies to fatigue.

Eating "nature's most perfect food" can make you sick. Bee pollen can cause life-threatening allergic reactions in some people, even though it's often promoted as an allergy cure. Some early warning signs include numbness or tingling on the lips or in your mouth. If you have any reactions to eating bee pollen, go directly to the closest emergency room.

Chitosan

Chitosan (KITE-oh-san), like glucoasmine, is nothing more than crushed crab and lobster shells. Indigestible fiber from the shells supposedly binds and absorbs the fat you eat before it has a chance to be metabolized. Believers claim that chitosan can absorb up six to twelve times its weight in fat, but it also decreases the absorption of the fat-soluble vitamins A, D, E, and K and carotenoids. As with other fat removers or replacers, folks who take chitosan will end up spending more time on the toilet than usual. A few studies done outside the United States show it may have some effect on weight loss, but no serious research has been undertaken here. Because crab and lobster shells are a natural substance that can't be patented, there is little financial incentive to conduct extensive studies. Like other products, you can label it a dietary supplement and go to market without FDA approval or review. Also, if you are allergic to shellfish, you can experience similar reactions with these supplements.

Cholestin

Cholestin (KO-less-tin), a dietary supplement introduced in 1997, blurred the already fuzzy line between food supplements and prescription drugs. Cholestin is made from red yeast that has been fermented from rice. Its main ingredient is a naturally occurring form of lovastatin, a synthetically produced compound similar to the prescription drug Mevacor. Previously, the FDA declared Cholestin an unapproved drug because its main ingredient is identical to the lovastatin in Mevacor. A Utah processor sued in federal court and won the right to market the product as a dietary supplement.

Cholestin can be purchased without a prescription, but the price is about the same ($30 to $37/day) as Mevacor if adjusted for a similar dose of 5 mg per day. Until early 1999, the only data on Cholestin's health effects came from China, where the rice-yeast extract has been used for centuries as a spice in dishes such as Peking duck. Two studies presented at the American Heart Association's March 1999 epidemiology and prevention conference showed that a daily 5 mg dose (divided into 4 capsules) lowered cholesterol levels by 35 points, or about 15 percent in those study participants with elevated cholesterol levels. Mevacor, in comparison, lowers cholesterol about 60 points in people with levels above 240 mg/dl. Both studies were funded and researched by the company that successfully sued the government.

Since Mevacor can cause dangerous side effects such as liver damage, it's suspected that Cholestin may also cause harm. Only about 20 percent of people with cholesterol levels above 240 mg/dl currently take drugs to lower cholesterol. That is due to fear of side effects, the high cost, and the possible risk of heart attack. Cholestin is a natural version of Mevacor. There is no reason to believe, without further study, that Cholestin is more beneficial or less harmful than the synthetic drug.

GBL

GBL, or gamma butyrolactone (GAM-ah bew-TROH-lack-tone), is an ingredient in a variety of liquid and powder supplements that claim to build muscle, enhance your sex drive, reduce stress, or help you fall asleep. Some popular supplements that include GBL are Blue Nitro, Revivarant, Gamma G, and Remforce. In January 1999, the FDA asked all companies distributing or producing products with GBL to recall them. Why? At least fifty-five people have gotten sick from this supplement, and it's been blamed for at least one death. Symptoms include seizures, slowed breathing, and a slowed heart rate. About one-third of those who reported problems became unconscious or comatose.

Glucosamine

Glucosamine (glue-KOSE-ah-mean) is an over-the-counter dietary supplement that's gained a lot of attention as an arthritis treatment. Glucosamine sulfate comes primarily from crab, lobster, or shrimp shells. Another less helpful version, glucosamine chondroitin, is extracted primarily from cow trachea cartilage. Because of its animal source, vegetarians may not want to use glucosamine. Sports physician Jason Theodosakis led glucosamine to fame in 1997 with his book *The Arthritis Cure.*

There's some evidence glucosamine may improve symptoms of osteoarthritis, but not rheumatoid arthritis. Osteoarthritis results when cartilage in your joints gradually wears away. Cartilage is the smooth, rubbery stuff that acts like a shock absorber so the ends of your bones don't rub together. You've probably seen it on the top of a chicken or turkey drumstick. The "wear and tear" on the cartilage is caused by overactive enzymes that break down tissue. Traditional treatment prospects are dismal: painkillers to ease the agony and, when that doesn't work any more, surgery to install artificial joints.

Glucosamine is what gives cartilage strength and rigidity. The supplements sold in stores are a processed version of the glucosamine found naturally in your body. Claims that glucosamine works by stimulating growth of new cartilage and maintaining existing cartilage are promising. So far, human studies on glucosamine have been small and lasted only a few weeks. Veterinarians have been using glucosamine since 1992 to treat arthritis in racehorses, farm animals, and pets.

Jane Brody, health columnist for the *New York Times,* reported that after she spent eight weeks on glucosamine, the osteoarthritis in her knees improved dramatically. "I do not have pain-free knees, but I no longer have disabling discomfort," Brody said after more than a year on the treatment.

Selected Studies

Ninety-three people with osteoarthritis of the knee were recruited for a randomized placebo-controlled study of a popular glucosamine chondroitin supplement. During the six-month study, those with mild to moderate osteoarthritis showed improvement at both four and six months on the supplement (American Academy of Osteopaedic Surgeons, 1999 annual meeting). This study, funded by Nutramax Labs, shows possible improvement for people with less severe forms of osteoarthritis of the knee. They received 1,000 mg glucosamine hydrochloride, 800 mg sodium chondroitin sulfate, and 152 mg manganese twice daily. No information is known on which single or combination of ingredients offers the reported benefit.

Royal Jelly

The thick, milky substance that is secreted from the glands of a special group of young nurse bees between their sixth and twelfth days of life is called royal jelly. When honey and pollen are combined and refined within the young nurse bee, royal jelly is born. Royal jelly is made only for the queen bee. It has no proven benefit for humans—even those with royal bloodlines. If you have allergies, be careful: royal jelly can cause highly allergic reactions in some people.

Lecithin

Lecithin is needed by every living cell in the human body. Cell membranes are made up mostly of lecithin, which keeps them from hardening or drying out. It also forms the protective covering around the brain. That makes lecithin pretty essential—so essential that it's made by your liver. You can get bonus amounts from foods including whole grains, fish, soybeans, and egg yolks. Most lecithin supplements are made from either eggs or soy products. You don't need extra lecithin and if you think you do, just eat the real thing.

Laetrile

Cyanide poison tops the ingredient list of the supplement laetrile. It's made from ground apricot pits and is still promoted as an alternative cure for cancer. Chronic cyanide intoxication from laetrile in the diet has produced thousands of cases of slowly progressive nerve damage. Common effects include muscle weakness, blindness, and loss of hearing. If you have cancer, laetrile won't help and will likely make you worse.

Fish Oil Capsules

Omega-3 fatty acids are the key to this oily sea supplement. Fish and fish oils have a great potential for the prevention and treatment of coronary artery disease. That's because eating fish or taking fish oil supplements works on many problems at the same time. Omega-3 fatty acids are most important in the prevention of arrhythmia or irregular heartbeat and can actually fend off the process that leads to many heart attacks. In addition they have an anti-inflammatory effect that *may* help to relieve the pain associated with rheumatoid arthritis and ulcerative colitis.

Try fatty fish first (e.g., salmon, mackerel), but if you don't like those, give white albacore tuna a try; it's about as unfishy as you can get and is still a good source of omega-3. If you choose fish oil capsules, remember you are also swallowing fat grams and calories. David Leonard, M.Ag., freelance nutrition/agriculture extension specialist, says, "To avoid possible contamination problems buy capsules labeled 'distilled' or 'molecularly distilled,' which assures that they are virtually free of PCBs, mercury, and lead, which tend to accumulate in some fish." A cholesterol-free designation usually indicates distillation, too. Capsules that also contain vitamin E and other antioxidants can help prevent rancidity during storage, but keep your capsules in the refrigerator for extra protection.

Pycogenol

Pine tree bark extract is the source of pycogenol (puh-KOJ-ee-noll). Pycogenol and other similar extracts are promoted as treatments for AIDS, arthritis, heart disease, cancer, Alzheimer's, attention deficit disorder

(ADD), allergies, and aging. Literature on pycogenol has been almost exclusively written by the product manufacturer. There is no scientific proof that pycogenol is effective against any disease or that it promotes health.

Shark Cartilage

Shark cartilage supplements became popular among cancer patients based on the theory that if sharks rarely get cancer, there must be something in them that could solve the cancer mystery in humans. William Lane, author of *Sharks Don't Get Cancer,* sparked public interest in this supplement. Test-tube studies in the 1980s showed promise. Harvard scientists found that certain compounds in shark cartilage have "anit-angiogenic" properties, meaning they block the growth of the tiny blood vessels that feed tumors. But the latest study, conducted by the independent Cancer Treatment Research Foundation (CTRF), tested shark cartilage powder on advanced-stage cancer patients; it neither slowed the progression of their disease nor improved their quality of life. As a result of the CTRF's study on shark cartilage, two new anti-angiogenic drugs, angiostatin and endostatin, are currently being investigated. However, no studies have been completed to date.

William Lane's son Andrew, now president of Lane Labs, which makes a brand of shark cartilage, says that it takes sixteen to twenty weeks for the cancer-fighting agents to work. Four or five months is a long time for someone with cancer to try an alternative therapy. With a cost of up to $1,000 a month, terminally ill patients might find a better use for their dollars.

Shark populations worldwide are now threatened because of the sudden popularity of shark cartilage. Unethical fishermen sometimes catch sharks, slice off their fins, and toss them back into the ocean to die. It's much more lucrative to harvest sharks for fin cartilage than for meat.

Selected Studies

A clinical trial at the Cancer Treatment Research Foundation in Arlington Heights, Illinois, provided shark cartilage supplements to forty-seven people with advanced forms of various types of cancer. After three months, five of the patients died and five had to stop the shark cartilage because of the toxic side effects it was causing. Twenty-seven people had their cancer worsen. Ten people had their tumors grow more slowly than expected, but that often happens (*Journal of Clinical Oncology*, November 1998). While such poor outcomes are common in people with advanced cancer, not one person had any tumor shrink or disappear. Since the research began in 1995, all of the people in the study have died.

Spirulina

Spirulina is a form of freshwater blue-green algae that has been marketed as a wonder supplement. This algae has been said to help with weight loss, improve the health of those with malnutrition, cure diabetes and hypo-glycemia, and treat addiction to drugs and alcohol. Those are pretty amazing claims for dried-up pond scum. The original source of Spirulina was algae from Lake Texcoco, a polluted lake outside of Mexico City. Most of the algae used in Spirulina are now cultivated in clean ponds.

Spirulina is a single-celled, waterborne algae that is rich in chlorophyll, just like all green or blue-green foods. Mainly it contains protein, which you probably don't need anyway. Spirulina also has some trace minerals, but you'd have to eat quite a few mouthfuls to get a reasonable amount. Even manufacturers readily admit there are no scientific studies that indicate Spirulina or blue-green algae has any benefit in humans. Why pay for pond scum that might be contaminated with bacteria, insect filth, and potentially toxic substances? Besides, it tastes terrible and may make you sick. "Cleansing" reactions such as headaches, tiredness, runny nose, constipation, or diarrhea may appear. Other symptoms, such as fatigue, skin rashes, nervousness, and increased susceptibility to colds, will supposedly pass after about a week, claim manufacturers. Often, customers are told not to use any medication that suppresses these symptoms and to avoid high-protein food because it can compromise the healing process. This is not good advice.

The next time you're tempted to buy a supplement that hasn't been scientifically proven to help, take your dollars to the produce counter or farmer's market and buy some of those more exotic pricey foods like mangos, papayas, raspberries, or red peppers that you might otherwise pass over because they're too expensive. The odds for improving health from nutritious foods are much higher than the chance that most supplements will provide a benefit.

8

Herbal Products

Do you occasionally drink herbal tea? Ever buy a jar of minced garlic at the grocery store? Sometimes add spices or herbs to foods you cook? Then you, too, are among the 33 percent of Americans who use herbal products. As you can see, surveys and studies that define use of herbal products use vague criteria. Consider these claims by reputable sources:

- Herbals are the primary source of health care treatment for 80 percent of the world's population (World Health Organization).
- One in three Americans, or about 60 million people, spends an average of $54 on herbals a year, totaling $3.24 billion (*Prevention Magazine* survey).
- Almost 70 percent of German doctors prescribe herbal supplements for their patients (Reuters News Service).

Such impressive statistics may leave those who haven't jumped onto the herbal bandwagon wondering What am I missing? Statistics can be misleading, so let's probe a little deeper.

It's true that a large percentage of the world's people rely on herbal or botanical remedies. Most don't have any other choice. Basic health care and pharmaceutical drugs are simply not available in many sections of the world. If you're poor and can't afford medication, you do what you can. That includes using local roots, herbs, and potions. Herbal products can be effective for a variety of conditions if used in the proper context. For many herbal remedies it takes daily—often multiple daily—doses over the course of many weeks to gain the desired effect. Herbs, for the most part, aren't a quick or easy therapy.

If 70 percent of German doctors prescribe herbal products, that leaves 30 percent who don't prescribe them. We're given no information on how frequently this 70 percent recommend herbs over pharmaceuticals—once a year, once a day, with every patient? In 1995, herbal prescriptions accounted for just 7 percent of all prescription medications covered by public health insurance in Germany. This figure sheds a little more light on the frequency of herbal practice by German physicians. Of course, many herbal products are also available over the counter in Germany.

HERB APPEAL

Use of herbal preparations in Western cultures began to boom in the early 1990s. You can now purchase exotic herbs and combinations of botanicals in retail outlets ranging from supermarkets to superstores. In 1994 the estimated market for botanical medicines was approximately $1.6 billion. Americans are expected to spend $4.3 billion in 1999 on herbal supplements that promise to do everything from lifting depression and shrinking swollen prostates to fighting colds and easing stress.

Time magazine's November 23, 1998, issue featured a cover story on the big business behind herbal supplements. Wall Street investment groups are now sponsoring conferences on how to buy into lucrative botanical medicine companies, just as they did with biotechnology companies a dozen years ago. Some analysts suggest herbal products will maintain yearly growth of 12 to 20 percent for the next several years. Growing herbs is big business, too. Herbs for health are grown in the United States for export to European and Asian countries. Currently, forty-three U.S. approved drugs are derived from herbs.

Where We Buy Supplements*

Pharmacy or drug store	32%
Grocery store or supermarket	23%
Direct mail order or personal sales	17%
Health food store	11%
Vitamin supplement store	11%
Club/warehouse store	8%
Health food supermarket	6%

Source: *Natural Foods Merchandiser,* February/March 1998
* Totals exceed 100 percent as some buy from more than one source.

Many traditional pharmaceutical giants have jumped into the market with herbal products just since 1997. They include Bayer (One-A-Day), Whitehall-Robbins Healthcare Division of American Home Products (Centrum), Warner-Lambert (Quanterra), and SmithKline Beechum (Abtei).

Top-Selling Herbs in the United States

	$ in Millions	Percent of Annual Growth Since July 1998
Gingko	138	140+
St. John's Wort	121	2,801+
Ginseng	98	26+
Garlic	84	27+
Echinacea	33	151+
Saw Palmetto	27	138+
Grapeseed	11	38+
Kava	8	473+
Evening Primrose	8	104+
Echinacea/Goldenseal	8	80+
Cranberry	8	75+
Valerian	8	35+
All others	1	
Total	663.4	

Source: International Research Institute, July 1999

Herbal remedies are appealing. Plants are living, fresh, and green—the very essence of natural. They might seem safer and gentler than synthetically manufactured pills. Using "herbs to heal" sounds better than "taking drugs." Drugs are perceived as negative because of their potential for harm and abuse. Why else would pharmaceutical companies be required to print all the warnings, side effects, and negative study results when they advertise their products? As with most debates, the issues aren't so simple.

Arsenic, nicotine, heroin, salmonella, and alcohol are all 100 percent natural botanicals and can be toxic or fatal, depending on the dose. The ancient philosopher Paracelsus summarized it best: "Everything is poison. There is nothing without poison. Only the dose makes a thing a poison." As with any nutritional supplement or drug, herbal products can and do have side effects. Botanicals are not inherently safer than other types of remedies. Some plants are harmless or beneficial if you use the berries or flowers, but the leaves can kill you—or vice versa!

From the dawn of history herbs have been known as medicines with the power to cure or alleviate a host of afflictions. The famous Ebers Papyrus contains an Egyptian physician's herbal remedies written over thirty-five centuries ago. The pharmacologic treatment of disease is grounded in the use of herbs. The coca shrub from the new world yielded cocaine—the prototype for modern local anesthetics. The bark of *Cinchona* species yielded quinine, a drug still important in the treatment of malaria. Salicylic acid from willow bark was extracted and refined into aspirin. Echinacea was listed in the U.S. drug formulary before the discovery of antibiotics.

Most herbal remedies do not give immediate results. This can be confusing for the many Americans who seek simple solutions for health problems. Therapeutic effects from botanicals often appear only after weeks or months of continued use. When you visit the doctor for something urgent, you expect immediate relief and recovery. It's the American way—"give me something to take care of what ails me and it better work fast."

We also want easy solutions—a pill to swallow just once a day—no injections, multiple medicines, or complicated dosing schedules. People with infants or toddlers are thrilled to learn there's a new medicine for ear infections to be administered just once a day for five days. Previously the cure involved trying to get four equally spaced doses of gooey pink medicine into a squirming child on ten consecutive days. The most common complaint from physicians is that as soon as a child starts to improve on antibiotics, parents stop the medicine. It's just too much hassle. But most herbal products don't have simple dosage regimens. Europeans and Asians are far more likely to take their herbal tonic as a tea or tincture. Multiple daily doses are common. Often it takes several weeks to notice any improvement. Herbal and botanical remedies are not simple, easy alternatives.

Herbal products are prepared in a variety of ways. Only a scant number of scientific studies have been conducted using herbal products found on American store shelves. When research shows that a particular herb is beneficial, there are many factors to consider before you buy:

What part of the plant was used?

What form of the herb was studied?

What was the marker or standardized ingredient?

What dose was taken?

How many times per day?

How many days did treatment last?

Is this product available in the United States?

How many people were in the study?

Who were these people and are they similar to you?

HERBS THROUGHOUT THE AGES

Source: Lichtwer Pharma U.S, Inc., 1997

AROUND 2000 B.C.

Emperor Shen Nung (2737 B.C.–2697 B.C.) published a medical treatise about the use of medicinal herbs. This was probably the first documentation on the subject.

AROUND 300 B.C.

Hippocrates, the ancient Greek physician known as the father of medicine, gave his patients St. John's wort for a variety of ills.

A.D.

Dioscorides, a Greek physician, wrote the *Codex Anicare Julianae*, an herbal formulary. He recommended St. John's wort for a number of ailments ranging from burns to recurring fevers.

Pliny, the Roman herbalist, prescribed St. John's Wort in wine for snake bites (A.D. 23–79).

The Greeks and Romans believed that St. John's wort's pungent odor protected against witches' spells.

St. John the Baptist, from whom St. John's wort claims its name, was beheaded (A.D. 32). The plant's blooms are yellow with red spots, said to symbolize the blood spilled during his beheading. It also blooms on June 24, St. John the Baptist's traditional birthday.

THE MIDDLE AGES (5TH–15TH CENTURY)

The Benedictine Monastic Order became famous for its expertise and use of herbal remedies. The monastic infirmaries were host to a broad range of medicinal plants.

The Doctrine of Signatures was adopted. It stated that an herb's physical appearance revealed its healing power.

In the Middle Ages, it was common for individual villages to have herbal healers. The concoctions brewed up by these healers have since been shown to have beneficial qualities.

Christians burned St. John's wort in bonfires on St. John's Eve to purify the air, ward off evil spirits, and ensure healthy crops.

Paracelsus (1493–1541), known for revolutionizing the practice of medicine in the day, embraced the practice of using herbs to treat and prevent disease.

16TH CENTURY

Numerous books about herbs and herbal medicine began to appear with the invention of the printing press. William Turner's *The New Herball* (1551) and John Gerard's *Herball* (1597) were the standard herb texts of the day and are still used today.

17TH CENTURY

Nicholas Culpeper, an English apothecarist, published *The Complete Herbal* in 1649. In it he wrote, "tincture of the [St. John's wort] flowers in spirt of wine, is commended against melancholy and madness."

Early colonists introduced St. John's wort into North America but found that the Native Americans used the plant much in the same way as it was used in Europe.

19TH CENTURY

Throughout the nineteenth century, homeopathy was as popular as "traditional" medicine.

Charles Millspaugh, M.D., a nineteenth-century botanical expert, used St. John's wort on wounds during the Civil War.

20TH CENTURY

Germany's Commission E was established to test the efficacy and safety of herbs. Many in the herbal industry tout it as a model to regulate the expanding herbal supplement market in the U.S. (1978)

U.S. Congress enacted the Dietary Supplement Health Education Act, more commonly known as DSHEA (1994).

HERBAL HODGEPODGE

Capsules: hard gelatin shells that protect a powdered or granulated drug. They also help protect the stomach and prevent dilution before reaching the small intestines.

Coated tablets: compressed tablets with a coating of sugar, dye, fat, and wax. The coating helps protect the medicinal core, extends shelf life, and can allow slow release of the medication.

Granules: mix of powders held together by binders

Lozenges: molded or cut shapes that can be sucked on or chewed. They permit slow release of medicine into the mouth. Often lozenges contain up to 90 percent sugar.

Oils: fatty oils or liquid waxes that contain solutions or extracts

Syrups: thick, 60 to 65 percent sugar-based liquids used to help mask the flavor of the herb and to extend shelf life

Tinctures: alcohol-based solutions with a limited shelf life. Popular "tonics" can be 50 percent or more grain alcohol.

Uncoated tablets: compressed powder or granules plus binders and color/flavor agents

Nightmare on Herb Street

The herbal marketplace is a regulatory mess. There are no federal standards for botanicals to ensure dose, safety, or purity. Many products are standardized according to industry guidelines that differ from producer to producer. Herbal products and botanicals generally don't contain calories, fiber, vitamins, or minerals. Therefore, no RDA or Dietary Reference Intake (DRI) guidelines exist for them. Herbal remedies are usually marketed for their "acclaimed" drug effect, but are not regulated as drugs.

The U.S. Dietary Supplement Health Education Act (DSHEA) uses the words "herbs" and "botanicals" when referring to herbal supplements. The more accurate term is botanical, meaning a substance derived from plants or a vegetable drug, especially in its crude state. Herbs, botanically speaking, refer to plants with a nonwoody stems that die back in winter. The DSHEA laws of 1994 forbid advertising that implies herbal products treat or prevent specific illnesses. But advertising, product labeling, and news reports still claim that "St. John's wort treats depression" or say to use "echinacea to prevent colds."

Right now there are four pathways to sell herbal products in the United States. A supplier can choose any or all of these distribution channels, each with different requirements.

1. Herbs can be sold as foods. You probably have some in your kitchen right now. They include flavoring spices (parsley, sage, rosemary, and thyme), candied ginger, minced garlic, jalapeño peppers, and more. Some of these products require Nutrition Facts labeling on the package, some do not. Only those that have significant nutrient value of basic vitamins and minerals must carry this label.

2. Herbal products can be sold as dietary supplements and make claims as to their effect on the structure or function of the human body. These claims are permitted as long as the company has adequate documentation. The FDA is not permitted to request or review this evidence. In addition, any product that makes a structure or function claim must print a disclaimer on the package: "This statement has not been evaluated by the Food and Drug Administration. This product is not intended to diagnose, treat, cure, or prevent any disease." Search out the smallest print on the label—that's where you'll usually find this note.

3. Some herbal remedies are sold as over-the-counter medication. This permits the use of more specific therapeutic claims—similar to some drug claims. This doesn't mean that the identical product can't also be sold as a dietary supplement, but it must have different labeling.

4. The newest regulatory category available for botanicals is through the Investigational New Drug/New Drug Application (IND/NDA) process of the FDA. Until recently only the U.S. pharmaceutical industry had access to this option. According to the FDA's Center for Drug Evaluation and Research (CDER), there are fifty botanicals or botanical formulas holding active IND applications.

Some herbal companies plan to seek Food and Drug Administration approval to sell their most effective herbs as prescription drugs. That way, doctors and consumers wary of unregulated supplements could choose, for a little higher price, a fully tested and regulated medicinal version. There already are scientific data from Germany that particular herbs have beneficial druglike effects. Germany's data prompted our National Institutes of Health to finance a study comparing St. John's wort to the prescription antidepressant Zoloft. The study is designed to determine which product will better help moderately depressed Americans. Such careful studies are new for the U.S. supplement industry, but more are planned.

Botanicals Approved as Over-the-Counter Drug Ingredients

Herb	Approved Use
Aloe (*Aloe ferox*)	Stimulant laxative
Cascara sagrada (*Rhamnus purshiana*)	Stimulant laxative
Peppermint oil (*Mentha x piperita*)	Antitussive
Psyllium (*Planago afra*)	Bulk laxative
Red pepper (*Capsicum* spp.)	Counterirritant
Senna (Alexandrian) (*Cassia senna*)	Stimulant laxative
Slippery elm (*Ulmus fulva*)	Demulcent
Witch hazel (*Hamamelis virginiana*)	Astringent

Source: *OTC Drug Review* Ingredient Status Report, September 1994

Why aren't more companies running scientific trials? There's little incentive to spend up to $500 million on tests that can take ten to fifteen years to complete. That's the process new drugs must fulfill. But unlike most prescription or over-the-counter drugs, plant material such as an herb can't be patented. Drug manufacturers profit only if they can patent the process used to create, isolate, or modify a drug. Competitors are not permitted to copy patented drugs. If a botanical company finances scientific studies about the effectiveness or safety of an herb, competing brands would be able to capitalize on the results.

If healing herbs were always as effective as the spin-offs patented by the drug companies, there would be no reason to produce pharmaceutical drugs. Many herbal products are not better or safer than pharmaceuticals. A case in point is aspirin (a derivative of the active component of willow bark). Aspirin is much gentler on your stomach and easier to swallow than natural willow bark. Both products work, but aspirin has fewer negative side effects. In *Herbs of Choice,* Dr. Varro Tyler calculated you would need to brew ten cups of the highest-quality willow bark tea to make the equivalent of a single aspirin tablet. If you substitute ordinary white willow bark, you'd need seventy cups to substitute for one aspirin.

Almost all synthetic drugs are first tested in laboratory animals before they are tested on people. Animal experimentation greatly speeds up scientific research and points to potential harm or side effects. By contrast, herbal remedy support is often linked to casual observation of what happened to particular individuals. Convincing evidence to support mainstream herbal therapy using U.S. products has not been completed. It's difficult to draw conclusions from studies of other countries that test doses and forms of herbal products not available in the United States. Consumers should demand, at the very least, evidence that shows which options are safe and actually deliver the results they promise. According to the Food and Nutrition Science Alliance (FANSA), too few herbal products list the contraindications on their labels to warn consumers of potential ill effects. Responsible manufacturers voluntarily provide this information.

DSHEA, which went into effect in 1994, prohibits manufacturers of herbal supplements from advertising that their products treat or prevent specific illnesses. Aside from that, the industry is mostly unregulated. Given the dramatic increase in volume and variety of dietary supplement advertising in recent years, the FTC staff has issued guidelines to clarify long-standing FTC policies and enforcement practices related to dietary supplement advertising. You're left on your own to find out what herbs are used for, how much you need, and what any possible side effects might be.

HANDY HOTLINE Call the FTC at 1-202-382-4357 to file a complaint regarding herbal supplements and advertising.

Germany is often praised as the world model for successful regulations and use of botanical medicines. The German rules permit herbs and botanicals to be sold either as self-selected or prescription drugs. Their government requires absolute proof of their safety and a reasonable certainty that herbs will do what they promise. The words "reasonable certainty" are extremely important. They require that some scientific and clinical evidence be provided prior to approval. These requirements are not the same as would be necessary for a new chemical entity. "Their system is the best because it encourages research," says U.S. herb expert Dr. Varro Tyler. "The literature is reviewed. They do trials." Because the German system is based in science, consumers are more satisfied and are guaranteed to receive a quality product with proven results.

That is not the case in the United States, where almost anyone can sell herbal supplements and claim they contain an herbal ingredient. U.S. consumers are largely dependent on the goodwill or integrity of manufacturers. Now that reputable U.S. manufacturers and trusted German supplement companies have entered the market, more reliable, science-based products are becoming available. In late 1998, the United States Pharmacopoeia (USP) released the first voluntary U.S. standards for the potency of nine herbal products. Manufacturers that follow these standards can add the letters NF, for national formulary, to their labels. NF is like the Good Housekeeping Seal of Approval for herbal remedies.

Buying Better Botanicals

You can't rely on health food sales staff or even pharmacists for accurate information about both the risks and the benefits of the herbal remedies they sell. An informal survey at the March 1999 meeting of the American Society for Clinical Pharmacology and Therapeutics in San Antonio reported that neither pharmacists nor health food retailers provided much accurate information on herbal products. For example, almost half didn't know any of the negative side effects of St. John's wort and valerian root. Since you are on your own when purchasing herbs, here are some tips to follow:

Buy "standardized" preparations. Standardized means that an herb has been processed so that every pill or capsule contains the same amount of one or more chemical "markers" (not necessarily the active ingredient). It will be listed as a certain percentage of the ingredients. Look for the USP National Formulary (NF) approval on labels.

Choose products that give specific and clear information on dosing. Don't use guesswork to determine how much you need. Start with the smallest recommended dose.

Buy from a reputable company that researches its products. Check with as many sources as you can to find out which companies are good. Supplements imported from Germany tend to be high quality, as do the newer ones from U.S. pharmaceutical companies. Find out what brands are being used in U.S. clinical trials by noting the journal source of published research and going online to find details.

> The *Los Angeles Times* commissioned a laboratory analysis of ten brands of St. John's wort. Three were found to have no more than half the potency listed on the label, and another four had less than 90 percent of the labeled amount. One of the lowest-scoring products, with about 20 percent of the labeled potency, was from Sundown Herbals, a division of Rexall, the nation's number-one distributor of dietary supplements. The other two lowest scores were from Pure Source and Futurebiotics (Associated Press, August 31, 1998).

Don't hunt for bargains. Budget-priced herbal supplements are typically lower quality. As more mainstream companies enter the herbal marketplace, prices will come down. In the meantime, purchase name brands you can trust.

Choose solid products rather than the liquid-based tinctures. Most liquids are not standardized. Many active ingredients are less stable in liquid form. Creating a *tincture* is a simple process of infusing herbs in alcohol, while an *extract* requires heating and greater concentration of the original material.

Check expiration dates. Since herbs are plant-based, they can quickly lose potency. It has long been advised to toss out any kitchen herbs and spices after six months. Currently there are no standards for evaluating the shelf life of herbal products. Choose products with imprinted expiration dates when possible. Like other medicines, store in a cool, dry place.

WHO'S REPUTABLE AND RESPONSIVE

SELF Magazine contacted 100 of the major companies in the herb industry to determine which provided top-quality products. Of the thirty-three that responded, only a few companies produce standardized extracts, have strict quality assurance programs that include outside testing, provide complete labeling information (including contraindications and warnings), conduct clinical research on their products, and offer comprehensive customer service.

Source: Adapted from *SELF Magazine*'s "Ultimate Guide to Herbal Medicines," November 1998

Common Myths About Herbs

HANDY **HOTLINES** for reputable herbal companies' customer service include:

Enzymatic Therapy 1-800-783-2286
Lichtwer Pharma 1-800-92-PROOF
Nature's Answer 1-800-439-2324
Nature's Herbs 1-800-437-4372
Nature's Way 1-800-9NATURE

Herbal products have been used for their health benefits throughout history. In ancient times, people used herbals because there were few alternatives. Knowledge about herbal remedies was carefully passed down until two to three generations ago, when Western medicine became the norm. Information almost reached the vanishing point in the rush to modernize medicine. Renewed interest in the 1990s sparked a response that was more enthusiastic than knowledgeable.

Although there are a variety of modern health care options available today, the use of herbals is growing. Herbs are now being used in conjunction with traditional pharmacological-based medicines to help maintain health. The benefits of herbals are just beginning to be verified in clinical studies, and scientists are discovering the key ingredients in herbs responsible for their beneficial effects. Nevertheless, myths persist.

Herbs can't harm, only heal. Some of the most toxic substances on earth are made from plants, for example, strychnine. The most common side effects of toxic herbs are quite vague and are similar to those acquired from drugs, the flu, or viral infections. You can develop allergic reactions, cramps, diarrhea, dry mouth, digestive system upset, headache, nausea, and vomiting from taking some herbal products. A significant portion of all currently used pharmaceutical drugs are derived, either directly or indirectly, from active ingredients that have been taken from plants. In spite of this fact:

- 80 percent of consumers think there is a low risk of side effects or problems with natural remedies.
- 84 percent rated synthetic drugs as having a moderate to high risk for potential side effects or harm.

Whole herbs are more effective than isolated active ingredients. Many herbs contain a variety of compounds, some helpful and some toxic. Many isolated ingredients from plants become mainstream medicines. They are sometimes safer and more effective when isolated. Penicillin is a good example. Obtained from a mold by the Department of Agriculture during World War II, all of its descendants are single chemicals made by the pharmaceutical industry. The vast majority of prescription drugs and many over-the-counter medicines are based on single chemicals. Most of these satisfy standards defined by the USP and provide the best control of dose, effect, and purity.

All herbs are the same—from my backyard or around the world. When an herb does provide some benefit, you need a standardized formula or home "recipe" that carries a consistent dose of the active ingredients that make it work. Wine flavor and quality vary from vineyard to vineyard, and melons from one field are sweet while those from another are tasteless. These same variations in climate and growing conditions affect the ingredients in any particular herb. Different species of the same plant may not have the same beneficial effect you desire. Some local co-ops or specialty stores may sell pure strains of herbs or seeds for home gardeners.

Herbs have been used safely for years—no testing is needed. The assumed safety of most herbs is a result of historical tradition, not testing. Testing is "a step in the right direction," said Dr. H.B. Matthews of the National Institutes of Health, at a meeting in 1998 where scientists demanded better quality control from the booming herbal industry. Matthews cautioned that the companies haven't yet proved that their testing methods work and there are no standardized tests. The herb industry is attempting to counter growing complaints about dietary supplements' quality and effectiveness by turning to science. There is a fledgling movement that encourages use of pharmaceutical-style testing to ensure you get what you pay for.

The doctrine of signatures has merit. This ancient belief states that the shape of a plant part determines its therapeutic value. For example, kidney beans are kidney shaped and should cure all types of kidney disease. Walnuts have a ridged surface similar to your brain—they should help with all types of brain disorders. These beliefs are unfounded and research in this area is unlikely.

The Western medical establishment is trying to discredit and discourage use of herbs. There is no conspiracy here—just a lot of ignorance. Most health professionals don't have the time or energy to learn about other systems and styles of caring for your health. After many years of formal training and daily practice, today's health care workers would have to completely retool their professional skills. Not only that, they are expected to set aside the scientific foundation of their training and adopt new treatment options based on testimonials and consumer demand. Some of the first U.S.-commissioned scientific studies of botanicals are just being released in the traditional method of peer-reviewed research publications. As more scientific verification of herbal medicines is available, it will be easier for health professionals to choose them as practice options. Remember, it's hard to teach an old dog new tricks, but it can be done.

Quality Products

The cup of coffee you make might be twice as strong as your neighbor's. The mix of chemicals in your morning brew depends on many variables: the type of coffee, quality of the water, kind of pot or percolator, brewing time, and temperature. This chemical combination changes if you make a pot of coffee at 6:00 A.M. and keep it warm all morning for refills. The many variations of this theme illustrate some of the problems of self-medication with botanicals. It's difficult to get a consistent dose.

The United States Pharmacopoeia (USP) Convention was established more than 175 years ago, when most medicines were obtained from the garden. Some physicians formed this alliance when they realized that the medicinal effects of extracts of plants, such as purple foxglove, varied greatly depending on how they were prepared. Differences in plant variety, garden soil, climate, method of preparation, and other factors produced a medicine that was far from uniform. The organization was founded to provide recipes and standards that would result in more uniform medicines having more predictable effects. Doses came to be better defined.

Dietary supplements are subject to looser standards of dose, efficacy, labeling, purity, and safety than required for medicines by the Food and Drug Administration. Only if harm has been proven can the FDA investigate a supplement.

Poor manufacturing practices are not unique to dietary supplements, but the growing market for supplements in a less restrictive regulatory environment creates the potential for supplements to be prone to quality-control problems. For example, the FDA has identified several problems where some manufacturers were buying herbs, plants, and other ingredients without first adequately testing them to determine whether the product they ordered was actually what they received or whether the ingredients were free from contaminants.

PROTECT YOURSELF FROM INFERIOR OR UNSAFE HERBAL PRODUCTS

- Look for ingredients in products with the USP NF notation, which indicates the manufacturer followed national formulary standards established by the U.S. Pharmacopoeia.

- Realize that the label term "natural" doesn't guarantee that a product is safe or free from chemicals. "Think of poisonous mushrooms," says Elizabeth Yetley, Ph.D., director of the FDA's Office of Special Nutritionals. "They're natural."

- Consider the name and reputation of the manufacturer or distributor. Supplements made by a nationally known food or drug manufacturer, for example, have likely been made under tight controls because these companies already have manufacturing standards in place for their other products.

- Write or phone the supplement manufacturer for more information. Ask the company about the conditions under which its products were made.

Source: *FDA Consumer,* September/October 1998

Safety Classifications

The American Herbal Products Association (AHPA) publishes the *Botanical Safety Handbook (BSH)* list of almost six hundred herbs and botanical products sold in the U.S. market. *BSH* has created a standardization of the safety of these herbal products by developing four classes of herbs with a grading for their relative safety and potential toxicity.

HERB HUNTER'S GUIDE

Here's a description of the most popular herbs in the United States that haven't been deemed dangerous. Some have proven benefits, others don't. Information from the *German Commission E Monographs* and the advice of numerous herb experts from around the world have been integrated into this section.

Astragalus

The University of Texas did test-tube studies that suggested astragalus may be able to halt immune damage caused by cancer and common cancer treatments. Human studies need to be completed before it can be proved. Polysaccharides such as astragalus are thought to stimulate your produc-

SAFETY RATINGS FOR HERBS

Class 1: Herbs that, when used appropriately, can be safely consumed

Class 2: Herbs for which the following restrictions apply, unless otherwise directed by an expert qualified in the use of the
described substance:

2a: for external use only

2b: not to be used during pregnancy

2c: not to be used while breast-feeding

2d: other specific restrictions

Class 3: Herbs for which enough information is known to recommend
the following labeling:

"To be used only under the supervision of an expert
qualified in the appropriate use of this substance."

The label must include proper information on the dose, contraindications, potential side effects, and drug interactions and any other rele-
vant safety information.

Class 4: Herbs for which insufficient data are available for classification.

Source: *Botanical Safety Handbook*, 1997

---

tion of immune cells, including interferon. Used frequently in Traditional
Chinese Medicine (TCM), astragalus is often added to hot broth. In the
United States it's usually sold as capsules or tinctures.

Standard Active Ingredients: not known, but choose products that contain only astragalus root. Other species such as locoweed may be toxic.

Dose: common TCM dose is 4 gm/day

AHPA Safety Rating: not rated

Cautions: don't use for acute problems such as high fever or inflammation. Not recommended if you have an autoimmune disease because there
is some concern it may aggravate your condition. Not appropriate for the
treatment of AIDS, cancer, and other life-threatening immune diseases.

Black Cohosh (ko-hosh)

A forest plant from North America, black cohosh is thought to relieve
symptoms of PMS and menopause, including hot flashes. Sometimes black

cohosh is also called black snakeroot. It was a main ingredients in Lydia Pinkham's Vegetable Compound—an early American "snake oil" remedy. Native Americans used it for a variety of conditions, including sore throat and rheumatism. How it works is unclear. At first black cohosh was thought to have estrogen-like properties; now that has been disputed by research.

Standard Active Ingredients: unknown

Dose: common dosage is 40 mg/day for PMS and menopause-related symptoms

AHPA Safety Reading: Class 2b (not to be used during pregnancy)

Cautions: in Europe it's not used for longer than a six-month period. Too much can cause severe headaches, dizziness, low heart rate, nausea, and vomiting. Studies suggest that black cohosh impacts hormone regulation. Toxic effects have not been studied.

Cat's Claw Bark

Cat's claw is a tropical vine from the Amazon forest in South America. It clings to trees with the help of hooks that look like cat's claws. The Indians of Peru consider "Una de Gato" to be a life-giving plant with many virtues. They use extracts of the bark for gastric and intestinal problems and for inflammation from diverse causes. It is also used against many types of infections, as both an internal and external remedy. They also claim that cat's claw can ward off diseases and cure cancers and tumors. It's also thought to normalize women's menstrual cycles and work as a contraceptive. Cat's claw is often used to treat AIDS, arthritis, cancer, and tumors because of its antioxidant and anti-inflammatory properties.

Standard Active Ingredients: not known. Cat's claw is widely available in teas; tablet, capsule, and extract form are made from both the inner bark and root of the vine.

Dose: unknown

AHPA Safety Rating: Class 4

Cautions: do not use if you are pregnant or breast-feeding.

Chamomile

Bright, daisy-like chamomile (KAM-ee-mill) flowers have been used as medicine since ancient times. Today five thousand tons of chamomile are cultivated worldwide each year. Chamomile is so popular in Europe as a cure-all herb, it's said to be the European's answer to ginseng.

Historical records reflect chamomile's soothing properties, but few controlled therapeutic studies have been completed or published that prove effectiveness. Much of the research available is based on one chamomile product, Kamillosan, sold in Germany since 1921. In 1987, German chamomile was named medicinal plant of the year.

The *Commission E Monographs* say chamomile is best used for "inflammations of the skin, mucous membranes, and bacterial diseases involving the skin, oral cavity, or gums."

There are no known side effects or interactions for chamomile, except for potential allergic reaction. If you are allergic to ragweed, asters, chrysanthemums, or related plants, you may also have a negative reaction to chamomile. Chamomile tea should be made from fresh herbs and should smell like apples. If your tea bag or loose chamomile smells like hay, it's too old.

Standard Active Ingredients: three groups of active ingredients account for the known benefits of chamomile; volatile oils provide a mild anti-inflammatory action, flavonoids help as an antispasm agent, and pectinlike mucilages help soothe the lining of the stomach.

Dose: 1 cup of tea made with 3 gm or a heaping tablespoon of chamomile, 3 to 4 times a day between meals

AHPA Safety Rating: Class 2b

Cautions: Do not use if you are pregnant or breast-feeding.

Echinacea

Echinacea (eck-in-AY-shia) is firmly rooted in America—the Midwest prairie to be specific. Nine species of echinacea are native to the central Midwest region of the United States. The largest volume of research has been done on the species *E. purpurea.*

This pretty, purple, daisylike flower is one of the top-selling herbal remedies worldwide. Echinacea gets its name from the Greek *echinos* meaning "hedgehog" or "sea urchin," because of the prickly scales of the dried seed head. It was first introduced into Western medicine in 1871 by H.C.F. Meyer, a Nebraska doctor who learned about its medicinal uses from Native Americans. Meyer made a "blood purifier" out of echinacea, which he used to treat everything including rheumatism, migraines, dizziness, tumors, syphilis, gangrene, typhoid, and malaria. Echinacea was a popular herbal cure in the 1920s and was added to the U.S. Formulary. Echinacea was quickly overshadowed by the introduction of sulfa drugs such as penicillin in the 1930s. In Germany today, echinacea is given by injection or applied directly to the skin. In the United States it is available in liquid or tablet form. Swallowing liquid is believed to stimulate an immune response from lymph tissue in the mouth. If that's true, powdered echinacea may not provide the desired benefits.

So much has been written on echinacea that it's challenging to separate fact from fiction. While echinacea does not kill bacteria, it does increase the number of white blood cells, which in turn can speed up destruction of invading organisms. Echinacea may also block an enzyme that helps infections spread. Its most popular uses are to help "support the immune system" and to treat common colds. As with other antibiotic-like compounds, you can develop resistance if you use it on a regular basis. Most experts who recommend echinacea advise you start taking it as soon as you notice the symptoms of a cold, and never use it for more than two weeks at a time.

Selected Studies

The first scientific test of echinacea in the United States was published in 1998. "Echinacea-Induced Cytokine Production by Human Macrophages" was the fancy title of a study that concluded echinacea stimulates the immune system. Enzymatic Therapy's EchinaFresh brand used in this study was standardized for a content of 2.4 percent soluble beta-1, 2-D-fructofuranosides (*International Journal of Immunopharmacology,* March 1998).

Standard Active Ingredients: *E. angustifolia* or *pallida* appears to be the most likely key, active ingredient.

Dose: depends on the potency, but usually 8 to 9 ml of juice extracted from the aboveground parts of the plant

AHPA Safety Rating: Class 1

Cautions: although it's rated a Class 1 herb, some experts discourage use of echinacea during pregnancy. Echinacea should never be used by those with autoimmune disorders like lupus, HIV, multiple sclerosis, or tuberculosis. Anyone with allergies to the ragweed family of plants may also react to echinacea. Do not use on a regular basis or you may develop resistance. Eight weeks is the longest you should use echinacea at one time, according to the German Commission E reports.

Evening Primrose Oil

Noxious weed—that's how this biennial herb is classified by many in North America. Evening primrose is one weed we transported to Europe in the early seventeenth century. The feisty, fertile seeds of evening primrose sailed uninvited across the ocean in the ballast of ships.

The special ingredient that the pressed seeds provide, called GLA or cis-gamma-linolenic acid (sis-GAM-ah-lyn-oh-LAY-ick), accounts for about 9 percent of this oil. A vast number of positive effects are touted, but not proven, for GLA. They include lower blood cholesterol, lower blood pressure, slowed progression of multiple sclerosis, PMS relief, and (saving the best for last) weight loss without dieting. Dr. Varro Tyler, in his book *The Honest Herbal,* makes the following analogy: If you assume that evening primrose oil works based on its GLA content, that's the same as thinking your "car will run better if the gas tank is completely full instead of only half full." If the GLA content is key, then two other plants—black current and borage—provide even higher concentrations than evening primrose.

Selected Studies

A 1990 study showed that any effect evening primrose oil had on PMS symptom relief was no greater than the placebo effect (*Medical Journal of Australia*, 1990). There is no proof that evening primrose oil aids in the relief of PMS.

Standard Active Ingredients: not known; some products are standardized for GLA

Dose: one 500 mg capsule, 4 times a day

AHPA Safety Rating: Class 1

Cautions: if you have arthritis, asthma, epilepsy, or migraine headaches, evening primrose oil could make your symptoms worse. If you take this oil on an empty stomach, you might feel nauseous. No data are available on long-term use and toxicity.

Feverfew

A number of clinical trials have documented the effectiveness of feverfew in reducing the severity and frequency of migraine headaches. Parthenolide in feverfew acts in opposition to serotonin. Serotonin is one of the most important brain chemicals; it lowers your tolerance for pain from headaches that involve blood vessels in your brain. Feverfew may also help by relieving muscle spasms in those same vessels.

The most common way to ingest feverfew is to chew fresh or freeze-dried leaves. But this can cause mouth ulcers and stomach upset in up to 15 percent of chewers. Tablets or capsules are also available, and the consensus is that 250 mcg of parthenolide daily will provide relief. The problem is that U.S. feverfew products are not standardized. Numerous studies and reports show that many brands marketed are of extremely poor quality. Your guess of feverfew content in any particular product is probably just as reliable as the label.

Selected Studies

- Two out of three feverfew products sold in Louisiana health food stores contained no parthenolide (the marker ingredient). It was not discovered if this was the result of outright fraud, failure to verify plant varieties, or adulteration of the product (*Journal of Natural Products,* 1993). It's buyer beware in today's marketplace.

- In a feverfew treatment trial, sixty out of seventy-two patients were determined to have fewer than the average number and less severe migraines over a two-month period. There were no serious side effects noted from taking feverfew (*Lancet,* July 23, 1988).

Standard Active Ingredients: Canada guidelines recommend a minimum concentration of 0.2 percent parthenolide.

Dose: one 300 mg capsule, 2 to 4 times a day

AHPA Safety Rating: Class 2b

Cautions: Do not use if pregnant or breast-feeding. May interfere with the ability of blood to clot.

Ginger

Ginger is a favorite spice in many cultures. It's the base flavor of many foods from curry to gingersnaps. Ginger has also long been used as a remedy for nausea and motion sickness.

Did you ever have gingerale to soothe an upset stomach as a child? Airlines stock it regularly to help passengers avert motion sickness. Ginger works in the stomach, not on your central nervous system. In fact, too much ginger causes the exact same symptoms it soothes at lower doses— nausea, vomiting, and gas. German health authorities have suggested that 2 to 4 gm of ginger is effective for preventing motion sickness. Ginger can also be consumed as a tea or in the form of candied ginger. How much ginger in a ginger ale? We don't know since the most popular brands (Schweppes and Canada Dry) do not provide information on the ginger content of their beverages.

Selected Studies

A group of thirty-six college students prone to motion sickness were given either ginger or dimenhydrinate (Dramamine) before being twirled in a "scrambler-style" tilted chair. Those who took the ginger twenty-five minutes before their ride did much better than those who took the traditional prescription medicine (*Lancet,* March 1982). Since then, three additional studies have confirmed these results.

Standard Active Ingredients: volatile oil 1 to 3 percent is the substance that gives the characteristic odor to ginger; oleoresin is the component that provides the pungent flavor. Look for both on the label.

Dose: 2 to 4 gm, usually in hard-gel capsules of 500 mg each. Take 2 capsules 30 minutes before trip and then every 4 hours. A 1-inch square candied or crystal ginger is approximately 500 mg.

AHPA Safety Rating: fresh root Class 1; dried root Class 2b

Cautions: Do not use dried root if pregnant or breast-feeding. Those with gallstones should consult their physician.

Ginkgo Biloba

If you are young or middle-aged and have no brain-related disorders, ginkgo won't do anything for you. If you're aging and suffering from short-term memory loss, dizziness, ringing in your ears, or headache caused by decreased blood flow to the brain, ginkgo might be worth a try. It usually takes up to six weeks or more to notice improvements. If no improvements are noted after two months, stop using it.

The *Ginkgo biloba* tree is a living fossil. It has survived unchanged in China for 200 million years. In fact, it's the oldest surviving tree on earth. Ginkgo trees reach up to 100 feet tall and 20 feet wide. In the eighteenth century, a German surgeon, Englebert Kaempher, was the first Westerner to describe the tree by calling it "ginkgo," which is the phonetic pronunciation of the Japanese name. In 1870, it was brought to Europe as a decorative tree. Many American cities now plant ginkgo trees to help combat urban pollution. These hardy trees can withstand lots of environmental abuse.

The parts of the tree used in herbal supplements are the delicate, fan-shaped leaves, which are harvested when green. Since the development of standardized ginkgo extract in the past thirty years, it has become one of the most widely researched and most popular herbal extracts in the world. Ginkgo leaves are dried and ground and the active ingredients are then extracted.

Selected Studies

The *Journal of the American Medical Association* published a study in 1997 concluding ginkgo is safe and capable of stabilizing a significant number of people with dementia. Sales of ginkgo were reported to rise over 125 percent after the *JAMA* article was released and reported in the press. Lots of people dropped out of the study after twenty-six weeks. But more people on the drug continued with therapy compared to those on placebo. Researchers studied only a single dose even though previous studies indicated that some need higher doses. Improvements noted in people with Alzheimer's disease and other forms of senility included better personal and social functioning. It's also important to note that one-third of the participants in the study got worse. Ginkgo doesn't work as a memory aid for everyone. Since it's safe and there are no known side effects, it wouldn't hurt to try it for a limited number of weeks.

Standard Active Ingredients: The standard formula provides a potency of 24 percent flavonoids and 6 percent terpenes. The extract named EG6 761 is used in most research.

Dose: usual dose is one to two 40 mg tablets 1 to 3 times/day

AHPA Safety Rating: Class 1

Cautions: none known

Ginseng

Ginseng (JIN-seng) is the Oriental herbal equivalent of the U.S. one-a-day supplement in popularity. Many people take it faithfully every day to ensure good health. Based on the Doctrine of Signatures theory, the human-like form of this root suggests that it treats anything that ails you—and as an added bonus, it will spice up your sex life. Choice ginseng roots can retail for several thousand dollars.

Ginseng is a low-growing, shade-loving perennial tree in the *Araliaceae* family. Ginseng grows slowly. It usually takes six years before the highly valued root can be harvested for its health benefits. Ginseng has been used for centuries in Asia for a variety of ailments. In 1714, a Jesuit missionary stationed in China, Father Petrus Jartoux, was the first Westerner to write about *Panax ginseng.* After reading Jartoux's description of ginseng, another Jesuit missionary stationed near Montreal, Joseph Francois Lafitau, began searching for the root. His discovery of American ginseng in 1716 initiated the harvest and export of American ginseng to China. In the practice of Traditional Chinese Medicine, Asian ginseng is deemed "cold" and American ginseng "hot." American ginseng is often used as a tonic for the elderly in China.

Buying high-quality, real ginseng is difficult. A 1995 *Consumer Reports* analysis of ten brands of ginseng showed a huge variation in the amount of active ingredient in each brand. They measured how much of six marker ginsenosides were in each brand. Some supplements had ten or twenty times as much active ingredient as others and one had very little at all. Two earlier surveys of ginseng analyzed a combination of fifty-four products. They found that 60 percent had levels so low as to be useless and 25 percent of the products had no ginseng in them at all.

Standard Active Ingredients: look for an extract standardized for gin-senoside content.

Dose: capsules of 250 mg/day of whole root or ½ teaspoon prepared as tea

AHPA Safety Rating: Asian root (*Panax ginseng*) Class 2d; Siberian root (*Eleutherocossus senticosus*) Class 1

Cautions: Asian root should not be used by people with high blood pressure. Ginseng can cause insomnia, diarrhea, skin eruptions, and the jitters in sensitive individuals. Make sure you get what you pay for; buy only from reputable manufacturers.

Hawthorn

Hawthorn is a thorny European tree with bright red berries. Flavonoids are thought to be the main active agents found in both the leaves and the berries of this plant. Hawthorn has been used as an early treatment for heart disease. It dilates blood vessels and can help lower blood pressure. As hawthorn relaxes and dilates smooth muscles in the heart vessels, it improves blood flow to the heart. Hawthorn also may increase the pumping action of the heart and help some people avoid chest pain. These actions are the result of prolonged use and are not at all helpful for sudden heart or chest pain. Heart disease is serious stuff, however, so before you try hawthorn or any other herbal product, consult with your cardiologist.

Standard Active Ingredients: a standard formula should contain between 5 mg flavone or 10 to 20 mg of total flavonoids.

Dose: 160 to 190 mg per day of the crude water and alcohol extract

AHPA Safety Rating: Class 2d

Cautions: this herb is not recommended in the United States because you can't buy a standardized product. Heart disease is a serious health problem; don't self-medicate with hawthorn. If you have leg swelling, radiating chest pain, or respiratory distress, see your physician.

Horse Chestnut Seed Extract

The dried seeds of the horse chestnut tree may help you improve the look and feel of those awful vericose veins. Horse chestnut seed extract may help control leg swelling, improve blood flow to the heart, and improve the overall condition of the veins themselves. Some research suggests it's effective as a treatment for chronic venous insufficiency (CVI). CVI causes leg pain, sensation of heaviness in the legs, night leg cramps, and swollen legs.

Selected Studies

A study of 240 people with CVI concluded that horse chestnut seed extract was as effective as compression stocking therapy in reducing leg swelling (*Lancet,* 1996). Horse chestnut seed extract worked better than nothing, and had the same results as an external treatment. CVI is a serious health threat. Any treatments should be conducted under medical supervision.

Standard Active Ingredients: look for standard formulas that have 5 percent saponins and 16 to 20 percent triterpene glycosides

Dose: 600 mg of horse chestnut extract = 100 mg/day aescin, usually in a time-release form

AHPA Safety Rating: Class 2b

Cautions: do not use if pregnant or breast-feeding.

Kava

Need a feel-good drug? Mellow out with kava (KAH-va), a member of the pepper family native to the South Pacific Islands. You might say kava helps induce a "don't worry—be happy" philosophy. South Pacific Islanders reportedly drink kava brews nightly to relax.

Kava roots contain a fatlike compound called kavalactone, which is said to have antianxiety effects and may also aid muscle relaxation. Some experts believe that kava interferes with certain anesthetics. German studies have shown it comparable to standard antianxiety drugs. Kava is not believed to be addictive. Studies show it takes about eight weeks of daily use to produce optimal effects.

A 1991 German study concluded that kava did not impair driving ability. However, a 1990 Commission E study said that it can affect motor reflexes and judgment for driving or operating heavy machinery. That may explain the report in the August 1998 edition of the University of California at Berkeley *Wellness Letter* of a Utah driver who had downed sixteen cups of a kava beverage and was arrested for driving while intoxicated. The man was driving erratically, even though his blood alcohol level was zero.

Standard Active Ingredients: only extract-based products are considered medicinal. Dried herb should contain 3.5 percent kavapyrones.

Dose: 60 to 120 mg of kavapyrones daily for no longer than 3 months

AHPA Safety Rating: Class 2d

Cautions: do not use if pregnant or breast-feeding. Do not use if you are taking antidepressants or other antianxiety medications or herbs. Use caution when driving or operating equipment; do not take with alcohol or barbiturate drugs. Side effects may include an upset stomach and scaly skin breakouts. Chewing a piece of kava rhizome can increase saliva production in your mouth and make your tongue numb. Chronic abuse can cause serious skin eruptions and yellow discolor of skin, hair, and nails.

Licorice

Millions of pounds of licorice are imported to the United States each year. Even though glycyrrhizin (licorice's active ingredient) is fifty times sweeter than sugar, you won't find the bulk of it at the candy counter. Almost 90 percent of the licorice we use ends up in cigarettes, cigars, and pipe tobacco to provide flavor and aroma. The rest is used in a variety of pharmaceutical products like throat lozenges. Most licorice candy in the United States is flavored with anise oil and doesn't contain a speck of real licorice.

Medical journals warehouse a variety of colorful case reports of problems with people who overindulged in the real thing. Whether you consume licorice candy or chewing tobacco laced with licorice paste, too much is toxic. Side effects include headache, fatigue, fluid retention, high blood pressure, or heart failure. Licorice, in small doses, has proven useful in the treatment of peptic ulcers, but careful medical monitoring is required. Licorice is also effective as an expectorant as it stimulates mucus secretion.

Standard Active Ingredient: 4 percent glycyrrhizin

Dose: 1 to 2 grams dried root taken 1 to 2 times a day, 200 to 600 mg glycyrrhizin

AHPA Safety Rating: Class 2b, 2c, and 2d

Cautions: do not use if pregnant or breast-feeding. People with diabetes, high blood pressure, liver disease, and kidney disease should avoid licorice-containing products.

St. John's Wort

St. John's wort is an aromatic perennial herb with golden yellow flowers. It is found in dry, gravelly soil in sunny areas and is native to Europe, but is also found in the United States. Its leaves and flowers, which are both used in herbal supplements, contain glands that release a red oil when pinched.

St. John's wort has been used to improve mood since the time of the ancient Greeks. Its name is derived from its flowers, which are particularly abundant on June 24, the celebrated birthday of St. John the Baptist. The herb is also named for the red spots that appear on its leaves on the anniversary of St. John the Baptist's beheading. "Wort" is Old English for root, herb, or plant.

Depression affects up to 20 percent of the world population, according to some epidemiological studies. As many as 5 percent of humans suffer with severe depression. Untreated, depressive episodes usually last for six to nine months. Depression peaks at around age 50.

St. John's wort is not more effective than conventional antidepressants. The advantage is that St. John's wort appears to have fewer negative side effects than prescription antidepressants. Unlike the tricyclic antidepressants Prozac and Zoloft, only 3 percent of St. John's wort users reported side effects (decreased sex drive, lethargy) compared with 10 to 25 percent of the synthetic drug users. It takes several weeks of multiple daily doses to generate a therapeutic effect.

Standard Active Ingredients: not known. Hypericin was believed to be an active ingredient, but that has recently been disputed. Newer formulas standardize for hyperformatum, but that hasn't been proven either.

Dose: 300 to 900 mg/day of a high-quality extract

AHPA Safety Rating: Class 2d

Caution: photosensitivity in fair-skinned people

Saw Palmetto

Men who reach middle age (40 to 50) experience a change sometimes called the male midlife crisis. And guess what? It's a hormonal episode similar to menopause, but with very different results. Some women might describe this change as a man's need to be seen driving a red convertible, preferably with a younger woman in the passenger seat. Of course, there's no scientific research to back up that theory. However, half of all men you know over 50 have benign prostatic hyperplasia (BPH). Changing hormones stimulate growth of prostate tissue that pinches off the urethra and causes a variety of side effects. Common problems include suddenly needing to urinate, trouble getting the urine stream started, urinary dribbling, and waking one or more times at night to urinate. Until recently the only treatment was a much-dreaded surgery, transurethral resection of the prostate (TURP). TURP provides relief from the symptoms but carries a small risk of incontinence, erection impairment, or loss of the ability to ejaculate—not the kind of stakes many men are willing to gamble on.

Advertisements that claim saw palmetto can "treat or prevent benign prostatic hyperplasia (BPH), prostatitis, and urinary difficulty in men" have encouraged many men to self-medicate. There's quite a long history linking this tropical plant and urinary conditions. Saw palmetto is one of five plant extracts that was used in 1500 B.C. in Egypt to treat urethral obstruction. Florida's Seminole Indians used saw palmetto berries for maintaining the health of their prostate glands 500 years ago. Saw palmetto was also used frequently in the early twentieth century as a mild diuretic and for healthy prostate function.

Saw palmetto is a fan palm of the family *Arecaceae,* which grows up to ten feet tall. It has clustered leaves, each with twenty or more thin-leaf blades with sharp pointy ends. The saw palmetto palm produces dark red or brown berries. The berries, fresh or partially dried, are the part of the plant used in herbal supplements. Saw palmetto grows in the wild in the United States, from South Carolina to Florida and around the Gulf of Mexico to Texas.

Active ingredients in the berries slow down the conversion of testosterone into a more active form. It's the active testosterone form that causes the prostate to enlarge. Over-the-counter drugs to treat BPH, including saw palmetto, have been banned in the United States because they were deemed to be potent drugs. Because manufacturers position saw palmetto as a supplement, it is exempt from the ban.

No long-term trials have been completed testing saw palmetto for BPH. Most men were studied for just one to three months. At this time there are no known side effects, with one dangerous exception. A newer blood test called PSA has helped increase the early detection rate of prostate cancer. Like the drug Proscar, if you use saw palmetto for six to twelve months or longer you can invalidate the results of the PSA test. Saw palmetto can lower PSA levels, which makes it much more difficult to make a clinical diagnosis of prostate cancer. If prostate cancer is not detected early, the prognosis is poor. See your doctor first to rule out cancer. Prostate cancer is the most commonly diagnosed cancer in American men.

Selected Studies

A meta-analysis that combined data from eighteen well-conducted research trials of three thousand men with moderate BPH found that saw palmetto used alone or in combination with other herbs is better at reducing the growth of excess prostate tissue than a placebo, and equal in effectiveness to the prescription drug Proscar (*Journal of the American Medical Association,* November 1998). If you want to use saw palmetto, get a PSA test first and talk to your doctor before you proceed.

Standard Active Ingredients: fatty acids, linoleic acid, linolenic acid, lauric acid, and ethyl esters are thought to be active agents.

Dose: most research indicates a saw palmetto extract of 320 mg/day provides relief.

AHPA Safety Rating: Class 1

Cautions: get a baseline PSA level before using this herbal remedy. Your doctor's ability to detect prostate cancer by PSA is diminished when you take saw palmetto.

Valerian

Need help sleeping? Imagine closing your eyes and opening a door to the odor of a closet full of old socks and pungent cheese. Valerian (va-LAIR-ee-in) doesn't quite qualify as aromatherapy, but it does have a mild sedating or tranquilizing effect. Like many herbs, no one has yet discovered exactly how it works. It probably depresses the brain centers and relaxes smooth muscles, which in turn helps you to relax. Traditionally taken as a tea, you can avoid the smelly scent by taking valerian in other forms.

There are more than 250 species of valerian worldwide. Most experts recommend the European form, *Valeriana officinalis,* because Mexican or Indian varieties can cause toxic side effects. Valerian appears to be so effective that it's sometimes used to break addictions to sleeping pills. The French buy more than fifty tons a year of this non–habit-forming sleep aid. It may take several weeks of continued use to help promote more natural sleep. There is no known risk of dependence or adverse side effects. Valerian does not work like a typical, instant-acting sleep aid. This may be an advantage since instant effects promote dependency. Use it for four weeks before assessing the effects.

Selected Studies
A double-blind, placebo-controlled study of 121 people with significant sleep problems showed that over time, valerian helped much more than diazepam and three other herbal preparations (*Psychopharmakotherapien,* 1996). At first there was little effect on sleep but a general improvement in mood. This confirms the notion that herbs often take weeks to show their full effects.

Standard Active Ingredients: unknown, but thought to be a combination of volatile oils found in the root portions of cut, dried plants.

Dose: 2 to 3 gm of the dried herb as a tea, once to several times a day; or 600 mg of the ethanol extract 2 hours before bedtime

AHPA Safety Rating: Class 1

Cautions: only the European variety (*Valerian officinalis*) is for medicinal use; Mexican or Indian valerian can cause toxic effects. All varieties may cause mild stomach upset.

LINK UP to http://www.rt66.com/hrbmoore/HOMEPAGE/HomePage.html to see Michael Moore's site featuring a collection of medicinal plant images.

Herbal Chips are for Dips

Sales of Robert's American Gourmet foods were up over 300 percent in 1998. Why? They sell snack chips coated with echinacea, St. John's wort, and ginkgo biloba. Sprayed-on versions of these herbs provide no benefit other than lightening your wallet. It takes weeks of daily, regular use for potential improvements to occur from most herbal supplements.

Herbal Tea Time

Herbal teas have been enjoyed for centuries throughout the world. It's only been in the last twenty years that they've become popular in America. Herbal teas are now commonly sold in supermarkets, coffee houses, and restaurants. Most are harmless, but not healing to drink.

Herbal teas are not recommended for infants and children. Both the Nutritional Committee of the German Society of Pediatrics and most major U.S. health organizations recommend no additional fluids (herbal or otherwise) for healthy breast-fed or bottle-fed infants. Water may be given as a thirst quencher during hot summer days. Fever and diarrhea are the exceptions where additional fluids are encouraged. Children's herbal tea remedies, while popular, have received stunningly little scientific review. Because children are growing and building new tissue constantly, it makes them more vulnerable to supplements.

Weak chamomile tea and weak catnip tea have been given to babies with colic and children with upset stomachs. Parents tend to think of herbal preparations as less harsh than medications. However, there are no herbal standards for dosage and no valid data indicating safe use for infants.

Don't Do Diet Teas

Enjoying a warm cup of herbal tea is often soothing. However, specially designed "diet" teas that claim to promote weight loss in reality just make you sick. Diet teas can have dire consequences and would more honestly be labeled laxative teas. Herbal weight-loss teas work by causing severe diarrhea and dehydration. Sure, you lose weight fast—water weight. As soon as you start eating or drinking, the pounds pile back on. Common ingredients include diuretic herbs such as dandelion leaves, juniper, and parsley. Aloe, buckthorn, rhubarb root, and senna are also potent laxatives. Side effects, other than frequent trips to the bathroom, include severe abdominal cramping, diarrhea, and dehydration that can lead to potassium deficiency. Over time too little potassium can cause heart irregularities and even heart failure.

LINK UP to http://www.fda.gov/fdac/features/ 1997/597_tea.html for more facts on dieter's tea in the article "Dieter's Brews Make Tea Time a Dangerous Affair," from the *FDA Consumer*.

Herbs That Can Harm

Herb	Possible Health Hazards
Chaparral (a traditional American Indian medicine)	Rapidly developing liver disease—some liver damage may be irreversible; has caused at least six cases of acute non-viral hepatitis in North America.
Comfrey (KUM-free) contains unsaturated pyrrolizidine alkaloids that have been shown to be carcinogenic, toxic, and cause mutations in animals	May lead to death; has been linked to at least seven cases of obstructed blood flow from the liver with a potential for cirrhosis. Australia, Canada, Germany, and Great Britain ban or restrict availability of comfrey for safety reasons.
Ephedra (ih-FED-ruh) (Ma huang, Chinese ephedra, epitonin) contains stimulants found in some asthma drugs and decongestants	Range of effects includes high blood pressure, irregular heartbeat, nerve damage, injury, insomnia, psychosis, memory loss, tremors, headache, seizures, heart attack, stroke, and death. Several states have banned ephedra since it has been linked to at least fifteen deaths.
Germander	Liver disease, may be fatal
Lobelia (Indian tobacco, was used to treat asthma and bronchitis in the nineteenth century) acts like a mildly potent nicotine	Ranges from breathing problems, sweating, rapid heartbeat, low blood pressure, and possible coma or death at higher doses.
Magnolia-Stephania preparation	Kidney disease that may lead to permanent kidney failure; has resulted in at least twenty people needing kidney transplants or dialysis
Sassafras (removed from root beer production over thirty years ago, all sassafras bark banned from food use)	Nervous system stimulant, causes cancer in laboratory rats
Willow bark (may be marketed as an aspirin-free product but it contains an ingredient that converts to the same active ingredient in aspirin)	Reye's syndrome, a potentially fatal disease associated with aspirin intake in children with chicken pox or flu-like symptoms; allergic reactions in adults
Wormwood (contains absinthe, an addictive substance)	Can damage the nervous system and even cause paralysis. It also can lead to mental deterioration and illness. Oil of wormwood is used to flavor absinthe, a liqueur that is illegal in the United States.
Yohimbe (from the bark of an African tree, used for impotence or as a male aphrodisiac)	Overdose can cause weakness followed by paralysis, fatigue, stomach disorders, nervous stimulation, and even death. Some states have classified it as a dangerous drug that is available only through prescription.

Source: Adapted from FDA Supplements Associated with Illness and Injuries Statement before Senate Committee on Labor and Human Resources and *FDA Consumer Magazine*, 1998

PROFESSIONAL HELP

When it comes to seeking advice about herbal remedies, a 1997 *Prevention Magazine* survey found that people turn to friends and family, magazines, books, and health food stores more often than they turn to their doctors. Little wonder. Most physicians, pharmacists, and dietitians aren't well versed in the medicinal uses of herbs. According to a survey conducted at the Center for Food Marketing, St. Joseph's University, Philadelphia, every one of the more than three hundred pharmacists interviewed said they were queried about herbals by their customers but most were unable to respond to the questions posed.

Up to 25 percent of all modern pharmaceutical drugs are derived from herbs. Some of the more common include aspirin (willow bark); digitalis, a heart medication (foxglove); birth control pills (Mexican yam); and taxol for cancer treatment (Pacific yew tree). Today, few pharmacists and physicians receive any training in the medicinal use of herbs. They used to, but most schools dropped their classes about plant origins of medicine when high-tech drugs became popular after World War II. Despite the pull-back from professional training, pharmaceutical companies are scouring the earth's rain forests for plants that might deliver a new wonder drug.

The pharmaceutical industry has focused on medicines that can be produced in a laboratory, under strict scientific control. This standardization helps to make each medication chemically stable and consistent. That way each and every pill in your bottle will have the same amount of active ingredients. The question is, have the real active ingredients been identified? In the case of St. John's wort, products have been standardized for hypericin content. New research shows that hypericin is not the active ingredient. That standard was rescinded by the Federal Institute for Drugs and Medical Products in Germany. Current dose recommendations in Germany are now based strictly on the total amount of extract contained in the drug product.

Some herbalists argue that standardization changes the whole essence of a plant. In the search for the active components, some lesser-known ingredients that enhance potency or effectiveness may be overlooked. Maybe some plant ingredients help buffer toxic side effects. Transforming herbs so they are more like pharmaceuticals is a problem for some herbal enthusiasts. It's harder for people to deny they are seeking druglike effects from herbs when they are popping purified pills from plastic bottles.

WEEDING THROUGH HERBAL RESEARCH

The amount of information on herbal products for consumers is staggering. A proliferation of reputable scientific reference material on herbs was published in 1998 and 1999. Here's a sampling of titles targeted to both professionals and consumers.

German Commission E Monographs, Mark Blumenthal (American Botanical Council, 1998) ISBN 0-9655555-0-X ($189.00 hardcover)

In Germany, herbs are solidly mainstream. That's largely because the German government regulates them. A panel known as Commission E reviews the safety and efficacy of herbal treatments and regularly publishes the latest findings in an official register. Until now, U.S. physicians and consumers who wanted herbal medical guidance but didn't speak German were out of luck. In October 1998, the American Botanical Council published English translations of 300 of the Commission E reports in a large volume.

The Green Pharmacy, James A. Duke, Ph.D. (Rodale Press, 1999) ISBN 1-57954-124-0 ($17.95)

Written by one of America's foremost authorities in the field of herbal medicine, this book is an easy-to-use guide. Dr. Duke forgets, however, that some folks like to see references included, so they can look up information on their own.

Herbal Physician's Desk Reference (PDR) (Medical Economics, 1998) ISBN 1-56363-292-6 ($59.95 hardcover)

From the publishers of the classic *PDR* for prescription and non-prescription medications, this book aims to give doctors and health care workers unbiased data to guide patients who may be taking such alternative therapies. Each herbal product listed includes a review of available information on indications, pharmacological effects, proper dosage, precautions, adverse reactions, symptoms of overdose, and recommended emergency treatment. The *Herbal PDR* incorporates and expands on information contained in the original *Commission E Monographs.*

Herbs of Choice, Varro E. Tyler (Haworth Press, 1994) ISBN 1-56024-895-5 ($39.95 hardcover, $14.95 softcover)

Textbook format that provides information about traditional use of herbs, active ingredients, current clinical applications, safety precautions, and dosages. A nice companion to the *Honest Herbal* and includes more scientific background and information on how herbs impact a variety of health conditions.

Honest Herbal, Varro E. Tyler (4th edition, Haworth Press, 1999) ISBN 0-78900-875-0 ($24.95)

This book is probably the "botanical bible" for herb enthusiasts and professionals. Its conservative approach is firmly grounded in science. Few modern herbalists have the comprehensive background in botany, chemistry, and pharmacology that Tyler has. *Honest Herbal* helps you decide for yourself, based on the most recent scientific evidence, whether an herb is useful, worthless, or hazardous for a particular condition. Start here for the basics.

Rational Phytotherapy, Volker Schulz, Rudolf Hansel, Varro E. Tyler (Springer, 1998) ISBN 3-540-62648-4 ($49.00 hardcover)

If your doctor gives you a blank look when asked about herbs, try recommending a copy of *Rational Phytotherapy.* It offers quick insight into dosage, usage form, and effects of the most prominent herbal remedies. It may be the first comprehensive, science-based herbal reference book for physicians and health care providers written in English. It's based on scientific research including human clinical trials. Stuffy and technical, it's not an easy read.

LINK UP to **http://www.herbalgram.org** for information from the American Botanical Council.

Herb experts like Dr. Varro Tyler say these new resources mean that U.S. doctors now have unprecedented access to solid, clinical evidence of what herbal

LINK UP to **http://www.herbs.org** for information from the Herb Research Foundation.

remedies can do as well as which ones to avoid. "American physicians will no longer have an excuse to be ignorant," says Tyler. That's a relief, because the FDA urges consumers to check with their doctors when they have questions on herbal supplements. Even with a base of information now available, there is still little knowledge about how botanicals interact with common food and drugs. Most studies haven't looked at effects of long-term use of herbal products. Even poison control centers can't supply needed information on most herbal products.

Scientific support can't keep pace with public demand. Two major issues facing the industry need to be resolved. Hundreds of studies will not advance the science of herbal therapy unless these goals are met:

1. Admit that many botanicals are standardized on marker rather than active chemical components. We need to measure the substances that produce the desired effect, not just specific random components of a plant.

2. Develop industry-wide processes to analyze and identify the active chemical components and ensure a batch-to-batch similarity of products.

Future Focus

Up till now the major issues for herbal medicines have been acceptance and standardization. Other issues loom on the horizon.

Supplies of some plants may already be endangered due to sudden increases in demand. Most medicinal plants are harvested from the wild. Local people who hand-harvest small supplies for their immediate needs have little impact on the environment. Major corporations seeking large quantities for mass production may significantly harm fragile ecosystems.

Overharvesting of a growing number of areas is necessary to meet world-wide demands. A 1996 report showed that nearly 75 percent of the golden-seal population was vulnerable, endangered, or extinct. Pristine prairies on the Great Plains in North America are being decimated by "floral strip miners." Echinacea poachers dig out the roots of purple coneflower plants and leave the landscape pockmarked with holes, and little hope for the native flower to return.

Exploitation of indigenous people's knowledge of medicines, without the appropriate compensation. Often local communities help provide information about best use and doses of botanicals. Some herbalists suggest it's unfair to exploit this intellectual property without fair payment. Even the ownership of the plant material itself could be a problem.

Potential for harmful interaction. Many clinical trials are still designed without consideration of the unique characteristics of botanicals and how they may affect other things you consume.

Insurance reimbursement by managed care organizations has been increasing. Interest in the use of botanicals and partial coverage of their expense will probably be the key to their widespread acceptance.

Unique delivery systems are also emerging; for example, a St. John's wort skin patch, yam cream for estrogen therapy, sustained-release herbal formulas, or micro-encapsulated herbs that promote immediate absorption.

PART III

Healing and Hype

9

Eating to Heal

Over most of the past thousand years, the human lifespan increased only modestly. Since the start of the twentieth century, it has skyrocketed. The potential to improve health and cure disease will surely improve in the twenty-first century. On the downside, long-term research to determine side effects of new therapies can't keep pace with scientific breakthroughs. Most people don't want to wait for new "miracle cures" to go through years of scientific clinical trials. For example, Fen-phen and Redux weight-loss drugs were thought to be safe in 1997, and they were, for the small group of individuals in short-term research studies. When these drugs were marketed to larger numbers of people, the potential for heart damage first turned up. There are always risks, known and unknown, with any medication, supplement, herbal preparation, or other intervention. Perhaps the best question is: Do potential benefits outweigh the risks?

NUTRITION CONNECTIONS: DIET AND DISEASE

As medical and nutrition experts discover more about the connections between food and health, dietary recommendations will continue to evolve. In this section we'll review the top nutrition-related health problems today. A summary of the current nutrition issues that focus on each problem is included to explain how new research has changed our understanding and treatment. Selected research studies are included for health concerns not covered elsewhere in this book. In the *New Nutrition* recommendations section are specific nutritional goals and objectives that will help you optimize your health. Included are suggestions for changes in what you eat, foods to focus on, supplements, and herbal products that may enhance your quality of life.

Alzheimer's Disease

About 4 million Americans have Alzheimer's disease, which each year claims one hundred thousand lives in the United States. Experts estimate that worldwide, 5 percent of people over 65, and up to 40 percent of those over 80, have Alzheimer's disease, an eventually fatal deterioration of mental function. It's thought that half of all women over 80 will develop some form of dementia that shows up as a significant decline in intelligence and social skills. Alzheimer's disease is the most common form of dementia. People with Alzheimer's have characteristic brain features that were first noted by Alois Alzheimer in 1907. We still don't know what causes Alzheimer's, and no effective treatment exists to stop this disease. Because clinical tests for Alzheimer's are often inconclusive, brain dissection at autopsy is still the only way to confirm this diagnosis.

Recently, there have been some important advances in Alzheimer's disease research. Scientists discovered a previously unknown abnormal change in the brains of patients with Alzheimer's disease, called the AMY plaque. This new discovery may lead researchers to a better understanding of the disease and to the development of new therapies. Ongoing studies of the inflammatory processes of the brain point to the potential beneficial use of anti-inflammatory medication in treating or slowing the progression of the disease. Treatment trials of a number of drugs, nutrients, and herbs are currently under way. These include compounds designed to delay the onset of symptoms or slow the rate of disease progression.

Nutrition Issues

Good nutrition protects both the mind and body. Well-nourished people fight off disease more easily, and that helps stabilize mental capability, daily function, and alertness. Many people with Alzheimer's consume very low levels of vitamins and minerals, particularly vitamin A, several of the B vitamins, calcium, iron, and zinc. These substances are essential for the health of the body and the brain. Vitamin E can be effective in slowing the rate of brain function decline in those with mild to moderate cases of Alzheimer's disease. The mechanism by which vitamin E produces this benefit is not known for sure, but may be related to the vitamin's ability to protect nerve cell membranes from oxidative damage.

There have been few studies that have researched traditional alternative therapies. In one large-scale trial in the United States, ginkgo biloba (an extract of various parts of the ginkgo tree) was shown to slow the rate of mental decline compared to patients taking a placebo. The benefit was modest and the results have not yet been confirmed in repeated studies. Generally ginkgo biloba is used to improve overall circulation, memory, and concentration in the elderly. There are no known side effects to short-term use of ginkgo supplements.

Research shows a strong correlation between Alzheimer's and excessive amounts of aluminum deposited in the brain. There are also excess amounts of other nutrients like calcium, silicon, sulfur, and bromine and deficiencies of potassium, selenium, vitamin B_{12}, and zinc. It's not known if high levels of aluminum or any other nutrient are a cause or a result of Alzheimer's. Once-popular advice to avoid aluminum cookware is no longer suggested. More significant dietary and environmental sources of aluminum include deodorant and over-the-counter medications like antacids.

High levels of the amino acid homocysteine—already linked to increased risk of heart disease—is also associated with Alzheimer's disease. Researchers say it may be possible to ward off some cases of Alzheimer's disease through supplementation with folic acid and other B vitamins. In heart disease, the higher the level of homocysteine in the blood, the greater the risk of damage to the artery lining. That, in turn, leads to the buildup of plaques in the artery wall. In Alzheimer's, homocysteine may similarly damage the vessel linings—but, in this case, the lining of small blood vessels in the brain. This, in turn, decreases blood flow to certain brain areas, and may predispose some people to the brain plaques that characterize Alzheimer's.

In theory, estrogen may improve brain function by raising levels of certain enzymes crucial to learning and memory, stimulating the growth of brain-cell connections, and increasing cerebral blood flow. Five of the best observational studies, all done in the past few years, suggest that older women who take replacement estrogen may have a reduced risk of developing Alzheimer's disease.

LINK UP to http://ww.alz.org, the Alzheimer's Organization, for information for both patients and caregivers.

Selected Studies

A study of 164 people with Alzheimer's aged 55 or older had 25 percent more homocysteine in their blood than people the same age without the disease (*Archives of Neurology,* November 1999). Although it may be premature to advocate population-wide screening programs, you may want to add homocysteine levels to the battery of blood tests that are routinely done at your medical checkups.

New Nutrition *Recommendations for Alzheimer's Disease*

- Carefully monitor meal planning and eating. People with Alzheimer's need optimal nutrition and often are not capable of managing this on their own.
- Eat plenty of fruits and vegetables. Experts say eating a well-balanced diet with at least five servings of fresh fruits and vegetables per day is the best way to keep homocysteine levels normal. Dark green leafy vegetables and orange juice are also good sources of folic acid.

- Choose fortified whole grains. Since fortification of enriched cereal grains began, folic acid can be found in enriched bread, pasta, flour, cereal, rice, and other grain foods in the United States.

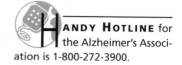

HANDY **HOTLINE** for the Alzheimer's Association is 1-800-272-3900.

- Check with your health care provider about supplements, to prevent interactions with current medications. For example, folic acid and B vitamins break down homocysteine in the body, thereby reducing blood levels.
- Eat smaller, more frequent meals to help increase food intake since appetite is often diminished.
- Engage in a more active lifestyle. Walk instead of drive, and take the stairs instead of the elevator. Sedentary lifestyles have been linked to Alzheimer's disease.
- Consider a trial of ginkgo biloba supplements for six weeks. If no improvement is noted, discontinue.

LINK UP to http://ww.alzheimers.com for additional resources and references on Alzheimer's disease provided by Alzheimers.com from PlanetRx.

Anemia

"Iron poor, tired blood" is a good way to describe anemia. It's a blood condition in which the number and/or size of the red blood cells is reduced. Because red blood cells move oxygen from your lungs to the tissues, any decrease in size or amount limits how much oxygen is transported. Common symptoms of anemia include weakness, tiredness, poor concentration skills, pale skin, mild depression, and an increased risk of infection.

A variety of events can cause anemia. Trauma such as surgery or an accident that results in a large loss of blood can make you anemic in a matter of minutes. Slow internal bleeding or long-term marginal nutrient deficiencies can cause anemia over time.

Nutrition Issues

There are three different types of nutritional anemias: iron, B_{12}, and folate. Having a low hemoglobin or hematocrit level doesn't tell you which nutritional anemia you have. A serum ferritin test is more sensitive for detecting iron-deficiency anemia, the most common type.

Women of childbearing age and young children are most susceptible to iron-deficiency anemia. It takes a long time for this type of anemia to occur. Infants whose mothers had poor iron status during pregnancy are most susceptible to anemia, as are babies who are not breast-fed and are given infant formula that is not iron fortified. Before menopause, women need almost twice as much iron as men do, because of the menstrual blood they lose each month.

It's hard for women and children to get enough iron from the foods they eat. It's not that there aren't enough iron-rich foods—there are plenty. The problem is that there are many obstacles to absorbing the iron from foods. On average, only about 10 percent of the iron you eat is absorbed. Your body is incredibly adept at hoarding iron. The less you eat, the more you absorb. That's why vegetarians do not have higher rates of anemia than meat eaters. However, this adaptation only goes so far. If you get far too little iron, you can't catch up.

There are two forms of iron: heme and nonheme. Heme iron (found in meat) is absorbed at a rate of 30 to 40 percent. Compare that to nonheme iron (from plants); only 3 to 4 percent of the available iron is absorbed. About 40 percent of the iron in meat is heme iron, but all the iron in plant foods is nonheme. Eating just a little bit of meat can significantly improve the absorption of all iron in a meal. "Meat factor" is the name of the substance believed to cause this effect. If you can't or won't eat meat, then the acidity from foods that contain vitamin C (ascorbic acid) can boost nonheme iron absorption.

Pernicious anemia is caused by a lack of the stomach chemical "intrinsic factor." You need intrinsic factor to absorb vitamin B_{12}. Vegetarians who eat no milk or meat eventually develop pernicious anemia unless they take supplemental B_{12}. Anyone who has much of the stomach or small intestines removed is usually unable to absorb B_{12} and may also need supplemental injections.

Folate-deficiency anemia occurs when you don't eat enough folate-rich foods. Low folate stores during the critical first few weeks of pregnancy are linked to an increased risk of neural tube defect (NTD). NTD is a birth defect in which the skull and/or spinal column does not close properly. It's harder now to become severely deficient in folate since all enriched grain foods have added folate. Alcoholics and others with marginal food consumption are almost always deficient in folate.

New Nutrition *Recommendations for Anemia*
For iron-deficiency anemia:

- Choose a healthful variety of foods, especially those rich in iron such as lean red meat and foods fortified with iron.
- Include plenty of foods rich in vitamin C when you do eat foods that contain iron. The vitamin C will help absorb more of the available iron from foods or supplements.
- Use cast-iron cookware. Tiny iron particles from the cookware are transferred to food and can provide a significant source of dietary iron.

- Keep all iron supplements in a locked cabinet, out of the reach of children. Accidental iron overdose is the number-one cause of fatal poisoning in young children.

For pernicious anemia:

- Get periodic lab tests to monitor B$_{12}$ levels if you are a strict vegetarian or have had your stomach or intestines removed through surgery. Injections of B$_{12}$ are occasionally necessary when levels become too low.

For folate-deficiency anemia:

- Start a folate supplement several months before conception if you are planning to become pregnant, to help prevent the risk of NTD.
- Choose foods rich in folate (fruits and vegetables) and include generous amounts of enriched grain products.

Arthritis

Arthritis is the common name for more than one hundred different rheumatic diseases that cause pain, degeneration, and inflammation of the joints. Osteoarthritis, the most common form, results when the cartilage that cushions joint bones deteriorates. In the less common but more debilitating rheumatoid arthritis, the immune system attacks healthy joints, causing inflammation, pain, and sometimes disfiguring joint damage. The cause of rheumatoid arthritis is unknown.

Unfortunately, there is no cure for arthritis. It's not surprising, then, that arthritis ranks second only to cancer in the number of bogus "miracle cures." Americans spend about $1 billion a year on unproven arthritis remedies. Though there is growing evidence that some nutrition remedies may be helpful, no one therapy can be expected to work for every type of arthritis.

Nutrition Issues

Forty million Americans have some form of arthritis. As the population ages, this number will increase to 60 million by the year 2020. That's one in every five people. Can a nutritional approach help those who suffer chronically from the pain, swelling, and joint stiffness of arthritis? There is some evidence that it can.

The single most significant nutrition tool in managing arthritis is maintaining a healthy weight. Symptoms of osteoarthritis often subside when excess pounds are shed. Rheumatoid arthritis is linked to overall poor nutritional status. The inflammatory process of arthritis changes your intestinal lining and reduces the absorption of some nutrients. Often the long-term medications used to treat chronic pain and swelling can increase nutrient needs beyond normal requirements.

Because arthritis symptoms come and go, it's tempting to blame foods for flare-ups. There is no evidence that any food triggers arthritis symptoms. A common diet remedy is avoiding the nightshade family of vegetables (eggplant, tomatoes, peppers, and potatoes). There is no proof these foods have any effect on arthritis. However, it's easy to avoid particular foods if you think they are a problem. But beware: if you eliminate any category or group of foods from your diet over the long run, you risk nutritional deficiencies that, in turn, can aggravate your arthritis.

Fish oils, from cold-water fish or supplements, have been suggested as an aid for pain management. Omega-3 fatty acids are known to have an anti-inflammatory action. Several studies have reported an easing of joint pain and morning stiffness and decreased fatigue with fish oil consumption. Symptoms reappeared when the large doses of fish oil supplements (2.5 to 5 gm a day) were stopped. There is not enough current research to strongly recommend fish oil supplements. Try to eat more fish first; it's part of a healthful diet anyway. Check with your doctor before taking large doses of fish oil, since it can affect blood clotting, and it may interact with medications you are already taking.

Preliminary research shows that a vegetarian diet may be effective in reducing the symptoms of rheumatoid arthritis. The research diet in one study consisted of no animal meat, more fish rich in omega-3, less fat, and more fruits and vegetables. It's not clear which component or combination of them was responsible for the positive results. If you decide to try a vegetarian diet, it is very important to make sure you are getting enough protein. People with rheumatoid arthritis tend to lose muscle mass, so those choosing a vegetarian diet must take care to get adequate dietary protein.

The omega-6 fatty acid GLA, or gamma-linolenic acid, may suppress the production of prostaglandins that trigger inflammation. Two studies have shown promising results from using one to three grams a day. Finding a good source of GLA is more of a problem. Evening primrose oil contains some GLA, but it's quite expensive. Check the label to determine the amount of oil that provides one to three grams of GLA.

The antioxidant effect of vitamins C, D, E, and beta-carotene may offer protection from certain types of arthritis, in a variety of ways. Vitamins C and D may help with osteoarthritis. One promising study showed a slowing in the progression of osteoarthritis of the knee when people had 150 mg of vitamin C (the equivalent of two 8-ounce glasses of orange juice) and 400 IU of vitamin D. Vitamin E has been shown to reduce pain and inflammation. Low beta-carotene levels have been linked to rheumatoid arthritis. Getting

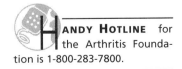

ANDY HOTLINE for the Arthritis Foundation is 1-800-283-7800.

adequate amounts of these nutrients, except vitamin E, is easy if you follow the recommendations of the food guide pyramid.

Jason Theodoskis's controversial best-seller, *The Arthritis Cure,* recommends using the dietary supplements glucosamine and chondroitin to treat arthritis. These compounds may stimulate the growth of new cartilage. Both substances are safe to use and have been shown to provide pain relief; however, it's too early to call it a cure. Clinical trials typically used a total of 800 to 1,000 mg/day divided into two doses. Several government trials are currently under way using glucosamine.

LINK UP to http://www.arthritis.org for the Arthritis Foundation for nutritional resources.

New Nutrition *Recommendations for Arthritis*

- Maintain a healthy weight. If you have osteoarthritis of the knee, losing weight will reduce stress on your joints. Every additional pound of weight is equal to three pounds of pressure on your knees.
- Eat a healthful diet. Include a generous variety of fruits and vegetables, whole grains, skim or low-fat diary products, legumes, and fish.
- Get regular exercise; physical activity helps strengthen muscles, keeps joints flexible, and aids mobility. Try activities that don't strain joints, like swimming or walking. Best of all, exercise can improve functioning without increasing symptoms. A lack of exercise, on the other hand, leads to weakening and breakdown of cartilage.
- Try cayenne from hot peppers; it stimulates blood flow, loosening up any blockages associated with stiff, inflamed joints. It also functions as a pain inhibitor when applied as a cream to painful joints. Devil's claw, used as a topical herb, offers relief by cooling inflamed, arthritic joints. Black cohosh is an anti-inflammatory herb and may also alleviate joint pain.
- Seek a doctor's advice. Getting prompt treatment can help to slow or prevent damage that might otherwise progress. Be sure to tell your doctor which supplements you take to prevent possible drug-nutrient interactions.
- Don't overuse nonsteroidal anti-inflammatory drugs (NSAIDs) such as aspirin and ibuprofen; they can cause severe complications like internal bleeding and liver and kidney damage. Check the package for information on the maximum recommended dose per day.

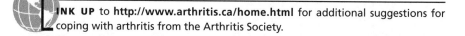

LINK UP to http://www.arthritis.ca/home.html for additional suggestions for coping with arthritis from the Arthritis Society.

Asthma

The causes of asthma are not clearly understood. In fact, there are probably a variety of circumstances that cause the spasms in the muscles surrounding the small branches of the lungs to occur. This constriction reduces the outward passage of stale air. Typical symptoms include coughing, wheezing, a tight chest, and difficult breathing. When the air can't pass freely to and from the tiny air sacs in the lungs, bronchial asthma occurs. These muscular spasms, along with mucus production, are brought on by histamine made by the immune system during an allergic response. Asthma often runs in families, indicating there may be a genetic link. Children who grow up exposed to cigarette smoke tend to have a higher risk for asthma than those whose parents don't smoke.

Nutrition Issues

A person who has any type of allergy may be at increased risk for asthma. Some children with asthma, who are also allergic to at least one food, may fail to respond positively to asthma treatment unless they avoid the offending foods, especially eggs, wheat, cow's milk, soy, and fish. Several sulfites in food products can also be a factor in asthma attacks. These can be found in preservatives for prepared salad greens, dips, precut or sliced fruit, coleslaw, processed potato products, and other prepared foods.

Vitamin B_6 has been studied for its effect on reducing wheezing. Those with asthma tend to have low blood levels of B_6. Supplements usually don't work to raise blood levels, but they may decrease the severity, occurrence, and length of an asthma attack. The antioxidant nutrients vitamins C and E, beta-carotene, and selenium may have a role in reducing the risk of asthma. It's interesting to note that blood levels of vitamin C temporarily drop during an asthma attack. There is no research to show why this happens or if taking additional vitamin C may prevent or lessen the severity of attack.

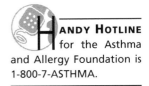

HANDY HOTLINE for the Asthma and Allergy Foundation is 1-800-7-ASTHMA.

Selected Studies

Overweight children are more likely to develop asthma than their thinner peers, says a study of 16,862 children between the ages of 9 and 14. In the United States both asthma and obesity are on the rise, but exactly how obesity may affect the risk for asthma is not yet clear (joint meeting of the American Lung Association and the American Thoracic Society, May 1999). This research suggests, but does not prove, that a large part of the asthma epidemic may be related to obesity. Researchers guess that obesity-related asthma may have a different cause from other types of asthma.

New Nutrition *Recommendations for Asthma*

- Maintain a healthy weight, especially in childhood.
- Take a multivitamin and mineral supplement in addition to focusing on a healthful diet rich in antioxidant fruits and vegetables.
- Consider 100 mg/day supplement of B6 for a short time (three to four weeks) to determine if it might lessen the intensity of your attacks.

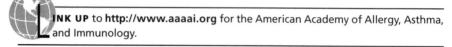

LINK UP to http://www.aaaai.org for the American Academy of Allergy, Asthma, and Immunology.

Attention Deficit Hyperactivity Disorder

Five out of every hundred school children today have been diagnosed with Attention Deficit Hyperactivity Disorder (ADHD). That makes it the most common of all child behavior problems. Typical ADHD children display fidgety behavior, excessive running and climbing, impulsiveness, inattention, disorganization, forgetfulness, and distractibility. Some studies have shown that teachers rate as many as 20 to 40 percent of the children they teach as having the behaviors that define ADHD. Most children with ADHD act perfectly normal when they are involved in activities that interest them, and learn best in settings that involve high levels of stimulation. These observations prompt some researchers to suggest that it's not the kids with the problem, it's just that they clash with our traditional "worksheet—stay in your seat" style of classroom learning.

There is much debate over the diagnosis and treatment of ADHD. In fact, there is no laboratory test that can be used to identify these children. The stimulant drug Ritalin was first used in the early 1960s to help control ADHD behaviors. Now an increased variety of medications and behavior management options are available.

Nutrition Issues

ADHD is a childhood syndrome that is recognized as an important medical-social problem and has been extensively investigated. Among the factors that can alter the brain function is malnutrition. Dietary factors could play a significant role in the cause of ADHD syndrome. Scientists are on the brink of exploring nutrition connections.

Dr. Ben Feingold started a revolution in restricted diets for children with behavior problems. The Feingold diet severely restricts foods containing salicylates, which are present in almonds, certain fruits and vegetables, artificial flavors and colors, and preservatives. You have to be fanatical to follow the Feingold diet. All food labels have to be read and investigated, making it difficult to plan and prepare appropriate meals and snacks. It takes a lot of time and attention from parents to help a child follow such a program. It's interesting to note that no scientific basis for these restrictions has ever been offered. However, a very few children do seem to improve on the Feingold diet. Two possible explanations seem likely. First, some children may have biological reactions or interactions with certain food chemicals or ingredients that can influence their behavior. Eliminating the offending substance will result in improvement. There is no harm in restricting food colors and preservatives, artificial flavors, and the few foods that contain salicylates. None of these is an essential nutrient or contains nutrients that aren't easily found in other foods. Every good scientific study of this diet say it doesn't work for almost all kids with ADHD. Your child may be one of the few who shows improvement, so it won't hurt to try, as long as you are careful to provide a variety of nutritious foods.

Since we don't know why these diet modifications work for particular children, researchers have tried to guess. The second explanation is that all the extra attention given to children on this diet is what causes the behavior change, not the change in food choices. ADHD children need much more attention from parents, teachers, and caregivers than other kids. When they get attention or are extremely interested in something, their behavior is more like that of other children. The constant involvement with food decisions may cause parents to spend more intense, attentive time with their children.

Promising new areas of research include fish oils and magnesium. It appears that many children with symptoms of ADHD have low levels of omega-3 fatty acids and the mineral magnesium and that behavior may improve with higher levels. We don't know yet if ADHD causes the low levels of these nutrients or if low levels increase the symptoms.

Selected Studies

- A study of fifty children aged 7 to 12 who fit the criteria of having ADHD and a recognized deficiency of magnesium were evaluated. During a period of six months, the children regularly took about 200 mg/day of magnesium. Hyperactivity was measured using various standardized rating scales. The children showed a significant decrease of hyperactivity compared to their behavior before the study (*Magnesium Research,* June 1997).

- A 1996 clinical trial compared the behavior, learning, and health problems in boys aged 6 to 12 who had low blood levels of omega-3 fatty acids to those with higher levels. The Conners' Rating Scale that assesses behavior problems, temper tantrums, and sleep problems was used to compare the boys. More behavior, sleep, learning, and health problems were found in the boys with the lowest omega-3 levels (*Physiology and Behavior,* April/May 1996).

- A Purdue University study found that fifty-three boys with ADHD had significantly lower concentrations of key fatty acids in their blood. A subgroup of twenty-one of these boys showed symptoms of essential fatty acid deficiency (*American Journal of Clinical Nutrition*, October 1995). The reason for lower fatty acid concentrations in some children with ADHD is not clear.

New Nutrition *Recommendations for ADHD*

- Eat a healthful diet. Include a variety of at least five fruits and vegetables, whole grains, skim or low-fat diary products, legumes, and plenty of fish.
- Give your child a children's multivitamin and mineral supplement that includes 100 percent of the RDA of critical nutrients. Nutrients that may enhance brain function include magnesium, selenium, zinc, and vitamin B6.
- Monitor height and weight at least every three months. Children on Ritalin or other stimulants may have delayed growth if on medication continuously. Some physicians encourage "drug holidays" during the summer to allow for catch-up growth. Experts believe that this delayed growth is not permanent. Instead of reaching full height at age 18 or 19, it may take several additional years for these children to reach their full height.

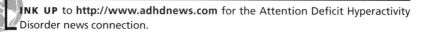

LINK UP to http://www.adhdnews.com for the Attention Deficit Hyperactivity Disorder news connection.

Cancer

Cancer has moved from second to first place as the leading cause of death in the United States, replacing heart disease. The National Cancer Institute estimates that approximately 7.4 million Americans alive today have a history of cancer. Scientists still don't really know what causes cancer to appear, much less how to make it permanently go away. When cancer does occur, it's the result of a mutated cell that multiplies out of control. When the growth progresses, it takes over vital organs and causes them to fail.

Nutrition Issues

Medical research estimates diet and nutrition factors can influence 70 percent of all preventable cancers and 35 percent of cancer deaths in the United States. In 1997, the World Cancer Research Fund and the American Institute for Cancer Research issued a comprehensive report on how we could slash cancer rates simply by changing what we eat and how much we exercise. Lung, breast, prostate, and colon are the four most common cancers for Americans. Smoking raises the rate of pancreatic cancer. Lymphoma and melanoma are both rising but there's no evidence that diet is involved. Kidney cancer is on the rise, too, because it's associated with obesity.

There is plenty you can do to cut your risk. The National Cancer Institute has made statements going all the way back to the 1970s about the role of diet in preventing cancer, but they haven't been well publicized. Sometimes people become fatalistic because they think "I've got the genes, I'll get the disease." People are beginning to understand that cancer is preventable despite family histories, just as heart disease is. But cancer is a lot more complicated. Unlike heart disease, cancer is a hundred or more unique diseases that attack different organs and that have different risk factors. One thing is absolutely clear: a diet high in fruits and vegetables is associated with a lower risk of cancer at almost every site on the body. This link with fruits and vegetables was not clear before the 1990s.

Alcohol is associated with a whole spectrum of different cancers. We haven't dealt with alcohol very much as a public health issue in relation to cancer. Not all cancers are linked to alcohol but decreasing consumption is important in breast, colon, and rectal cancer prevention. Alcohol, even in small amounts, increases the risk for breast cancer.

There's no question that gaining weight after menopause raises the risk of cancer. We know that hormones and reproduction have an impact because women who start puberty early or go through menopause late have higher overall cancer risks. Women who have children at a young age have a lower cancer risk than those who never have children or start having children after age 30.

Fiber is another component of vegetables, fruits, and grains that helps protect against cancer. Fiber does more than make stools bulkier. Fiber is fermented by the bacteria in the large intestine. It appears the colon needs some of the products of fermented fiber to function properly.

HANDY HOTLINE for the American Cancer Society is 1-800-ACS-2345; for the American Institute for Cancer Research is 1-800-843-8114; and for the National Cancer Institute is 1-800-4-CANCER.

Selected Studies

Scientists at the Arizona Cancer Center report that a diet high in calcium (1,500 mg/day) could lower the risk of cancer of the colon by 35 percent (*Journal of the National Cancer Institute,* January 1996). Researchers suggest that calcium soaks up acid that stimulates the growth of malignant tumors.

New Nutrition *Recommendations for Avoiding Cancer*

- Choose a low-fat eating plan that includes at least five to nine servings of fruits and vegetables and three to four servings of whole grains. No single food or nutrient causes or prevents cancer. A high-fat diet is linked to breast, colon, and prostate cancers.
- Aim for 25 to 30 grams of fiber from sources like whole-grain foods, fruits, vegetables, and dried beans. The protective effects of fiber are

associated with eating fiber-rich foods and not with taking fiber supplements. A diet that's high in fiber and low in fat may protect you from colon and rectal cancer.

■ Include more garlic and onion in your meals. The amyl sulfides they contain have been identified as providing protection against cancer.

■ Eat more vegetables from the cabbage family (broccoli, cauliflower, brussels sprouts, and kale); they contain the potent phytochemical sulforaphane. These cruciferous vegetables have been connected to a lower incidence of colon cancer, cancer of the esophagus, oral and pharyngeal cancers, breast cancer, and thyroid cancer.

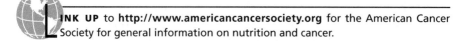

INK UP to http://www.americancancersociety.org for the American Cancer Society for general information on nutrition and cancer.

■ Drink a cup or two of brewed tea daily. Catechins and polyphenols in tea are powerful antioxidants.

■ Seek out selenium-rich foods. Selenium is found in seafood, meats, garlic, and whole grains.

■ Consider adopting a varied eating style that includes whole grains, fish, nuts, seeds, tofu, and vegetables; it's consistent with dietary recommendations for preventing cancer. However, macrobiotic diets of any kind should be avoided by people who already have cancer, because they may not provide enough calories and protein to protect against the wasting effects (cachexia) associated with the disease.

■ Trim all meat, poultry, and fish of fatty deposits before cooking. This will not only reduce your fat intake, it will also decrease your exposure to harmful toxins that are stored in fatty tissue.

■ Avoid foods grilled at very high temperatures or crisply blackened, especially fatty foods. The smoke produced by the burning fat produces polycyclic aromatic hydrocarbons (PAHs) that may be carcinogenic. You can reduce the negative effects of grilling by trimming as much fat as possible from meats, skinning poultry before broiling, and defrosting meats before grilling.

■ Reduce your consumption of smoked foods because they tend to absorb carcinogens that are similar chemically to the cigarette tars in tobacco smoke.

■ Don't eat salt-cured, pickled, and nitrite-cured foods (processed luncheon meats and bacon); these may increase the risk of cancer.

■ Limit your intake of alcohol to no more than one drink a day for women or two drinks per day for men. Too much alcohol increases your chances for liver cancer.

- Maintain a healthy weight and include regular physical activity. Obesity is linked to cancers of the breast, colon, gallbladder, and uterus.

LINK UP to http://www.aicr.org for the report "Food, Nutrition and the Prevention of Cancer: A Global Perspective."

Cataracts

The most common cause of blindness in the world today is cataracts. If you live long enough, chances are high you'll develop cataracts; in fact, two-thirds of all 60-year-olds have them. A cataract is formed when the natural lens of the eye, which focuses light and makes images sharp, becomes cloudy and hardens, resulting in a loss of sight. A cataract is painless and usually develops gradually over several months or years. Your ophthalmologist may prescribe stronger glasses, medication, or surgery depending on your symptoms, complications, or age. But wouldn't it be better to just prevent cataracts in the first place? Cataracts may not be an inevitable consequence of aging.

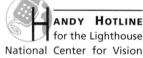

HANDY HOTLINE for the Lighthouse National Center for Vision and Aging is 800-334-5497.

Nutrition Issues

Studies on the relationship between cataracts and nutrition began in the late 1980s. Multiple studies have shown that increased amounts of dietary or supplementary antioxidants can reduce the risk of developing cataracts by up to 50 percent. Much of the oxidation that happens to your eyes is the result of exposure to UV radiation from sunlight. We're still in the beginning stages of learning which specific food components offer the best weapon to battle oxidation in the eye. One thing is sure: people who eat the most fruits and vegetables have the lowest rates of cataracts.

Vitamins C and E may protect against cataracts or at least delay their onset. Something in foods high in carotene also seems to have a protective role, but it's not the beta-carotene.

Selected Studies

- A number of epidemiological studies have suggested an association between cataract incidence and antioxidant status. A population-based study of 2,584 people from Sete, France, found that individuals with the highest blood levels of vitamin E had a significantly lower rate of cataracts compared to those with low levels of vitamin E (*Archives of Ophthamology,* October 1999).

- Results of the Longitudinal Study of Cataract Group that included 764 participants showed that the risk of cataracts was decreased by approximately

50 percent in subjects who regularly used vitamin E supplements and in those who had higher plasma vitamin E concentrations (*Ophthalmology*, May 1998). Vitamin E supplements are recommended for most people as they age. Here's one more study that shows the protective benefits.

New Nutrition *Recommendations for Avoiding Cataracts*

- Eat plenty of fruits and vegetables. Aim for a minimum of five to nine servings each day.
- Add blueberries to cereals, pancakes, yogurt, or just about anything. They are especially high in flavonoids that can help prevent eye damage.
- Take a multivitamin and mineral supplement that provides 100 to 150 percent of the RDA for the antioxidant nutrients vitamins C and E, and beta-carotene.
- Keep your blood sugar in tight control if you have diabetes. Fluctuating blood sugar levels can damage the lens of the eye.
- Wear a wide-brimmed hat and UVA- and UVB-protection sunglasses. While not a nutrition recommendation, eye protection is especially critical between the hours of 10 A.M. and 4 P.M. Don't forget to apply this same advice for your children; UVA and UVB light damage is cumulative.

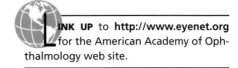 INK UP to http://www.eyenet.org for the American Academy of Ophthalmology web site.

 INK UP to http://www.ascrs.org for the American Society of Cataract and Refractive Surgery.

Diabetes

Diabetes mellitus is a chronic disease in which the body either can't produce enough insulin or can't properly use the insulin it does produce. Sixteen million Americans have diabetes, which is a leading cause of blindness, foot and leg amputations, and advanced kidney disease and a major contributor to heart attacks and strokes. Uncontrolled diabetes can complicate pregnancy, and birth defects are more common in babies born to women with diabetes. During the last twenty years, more people have died from diabetes than in all of the wars throughout the world in the last century.

For every two people with diagnosed diabetes, there's a third person who has the disease but doesn't know it. Because symptoms can be mild or nonexistent, many people realize they have it only when they develop one of its serious complications—blindness, nerve damage, kidney disease, heart disease, or impotence. There are three main types of diabetes.

Type 1 diabetes is thought to be an autoimmune disease in which the immune system attacks the insulin-producing beta cells in the pancreas and destroys them. The result is that the pancreas makes little or no insulin. Scientists do not know exactly what causes Type 1 but they believe that both genetic factors and viruses are involved.

Type 2 is the most common form of diabetes, accounting for 90 to 95 percent of all cases. It usually develops in adults over the age of 40, but is becoming more common in obese teens. In Type 2, the pancreas usually produces insulin, but the body cannot use it effectively.

Gestational diabetes shows up only during pregnancy. This type usually disappears when the pregnancy is over, but women who have gestational diabetes have a greater risk of developing Type 2 diabetes. Older and obese women have the highest risk for gestational diabetes. Children born to mothers with gestational diabetes tend to have higher risk rates for chronic diseases later in life.

All diabetics need to carefully monitor their blood sugar levels to prevent complications. Unless it's wildly high or low, you can't guess what your blood sugar level is; only a fingerstick test or blood draw can do that. Ideally, diabetics should check their own blood sugar level several times a day. It may not be too long before easier and less painful options are available. Several new devices are currently under review at the FDA, including an electronic inhaler that automatically delivers insulin deep into the lungs where it is absorbed into the bloodstream; glucose meters in the form of a disposable skin patch; and an infrared light scanner that painlessly interprets the wavelength of your blood and calculates your blood glucose level.

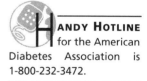

ANDY HOTLINE for the American Diabetes Association is 1-800-232-3472.

Nutrition Issues

Eating a well-planned, consistent diet appears to be part of managing diabetes for the foreseeable future. Diabetic diets have come a long way, and are now much more palatable and personalized. Here are the most common strategies to keep blood sugar levels in control.

The *No Added Sugar* plan has also been called the *No Concentrated Sweets* diet. It's pretty simple—no sugar, jam, jelly, syrup, honey, soda, candy, cakes, pastries, cookies, sweet fruit drinks, or any other food packed with sugar. This plan works best for people with borderline diabetes or those who simply aren't able to follow a more complicated system. It does not provide the best control of blood sugar.

Exchange Diets are perhaps the most familiar diabetic meal plan. Foods are categorized into groups that have approximately the same levels of protein, carbohydrate, and fat. With a dietitian, you plan how many of each group you may eat at meals and snacks. All foods need to be eaten in specified amounts at a designated time. It's a rigid system where food is in control.

The Total Average Glucose (TAG) plan is based on adjusting the amount of insulin you take to the total amount of glucose eaten in foods. "Points" are calculated from each meal according to its content of fat, protein, and carbohydrate. This approach is a good choice for very motivated people who need tight glucose control and who take insulin. The diet requires that you measure and weigh foods. It allows flexibility so that if you eat more or less than usual, you can adjust your insulin to accommodate the change.

The *Carbohydrate-Counting* approach focuses on the grams of carbohydrates eaten at meals and snacks, since carbohydrates have the greatest effect on blood sugar. Carbohydrate counting is more precise, yet simpler to apply, than the exchange system. You still need to refer to or memorize a list of foods and their carbohydrate content and must adjust the foods to fit your carbohydrate limit

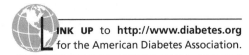

LINK **UP** to http://www.aace.com for the American Association of Clinical Endocrinologists.

each time you eat. This is the best option for people who are very carbohydrate-sensitive and need tight glucose control (sometimes called brittle diabetics) or pregnant women with gestational diabetes.

Exercise lowers blood sugar levels and can allow a little more dietary freedom. The best time to exercise is when your blood sugar is at its highest, which is usually about an hour after a meal. Active diabetics can have more concentrated sweets if they plan to engage in vigorous activity.

Artificial sugars have made life a whole lot sweeter for diabetics. Basically there are two types of sweeteners, those with calories and those without. The ones that do have calories—fructose, sorbitol, and mannitol—can cause severe cramping and diarrhea if you eat too much. That's your body's way of saying back off. Nonnutritive sweeteners like aspartame, saccharin, and acesulfame K don't provide calories or carbohydrates. As with all foods, moderation is the key.

LINK **UP** to http://www.diabetes.org for the American Diabetes Association.

Alcohol tends to lower blood sugar levels. If you consume alcohol you must carefully adjust your diet and medication. This should always be done with input from your physician or dietitian.

New Nutrition *Recommendations for Diabetes*

- Maintain a healthy weight; it is paramount for preventing or slowing the progression of diabetes. Excess body weight encourages insulin resistance, resulting in chronically high blood glucose. Losing as few as five to ten pounds can bring blood glucose down and sometimes prevent the need for medication.

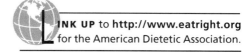

INK UP to http://www.eatright.org for the American Dietetic Association.

- Find an eating plan that fits your lifestyle. Work with a dietitian to personalize how you eat to maximize glucose control and your enjoyment of food.
- Choose foods high in fiber, ideally 25 to 30 grams a day. Fiber slows digestion, which causes blood sugar to rise more slowly when you eat carbohydrates.
- Do regular moderate exercise. This helps blunt the effects of diabetes in people who already have it. For every 200 calories burned in physical activity, vigorous or not, insulin sensitivity increases by almost 2 percent. The higher your body's insulin sensitivity, the more effective insulin is at removing sugar from the blood.
- Maintain a near-normal blood sugar level that is between 70 mg/dl and 150 mg/dl and frequently check blood sugar levels throughout the day. The Diabetes Control and Complication Trial, a ten-year nationwide study, demonstrated that by keeping blood sugar as close to normal as possible, people with Type 1 diabetes were able to reduce their risk of serious long-term complications by 50 percent or more.
- Do not rely on alternative supplements or herbal aids. None of them can cure or treat diabetes. It can be life threatening to stop insulin, medication, or your diet plan for false promises. The American Diabetes Association predicts a cure for some types of diabetes in the next decade. There are no cures today.
- Take a multivitamin and mineral supplement. Antioxidant vitamins may help mitigate the damaging effects of high blood glucose on cells and reduce complications.
- Check your chromium intake. There is evidence that some Type 2 diabetics may be deficient in chromium. Chromium helps insulin get glucose into the cells, so a shortage can mean higher blood sugar. Most Americans get about 50 micrograms of chromium a day from foods, including

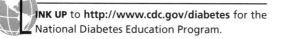

INK UP to http://www.cdc.gov/diabetes for the National Diabetes Education Program.

legumes, leafy green vegetables, whole-wheat grains, and nuts. The recommended safe and adequate intake of chromium is 50 to 200 micrograms a day.

LINK UP to http://www.onhealth.com/ch1/condctr/diabetes for the International Diabetes Center.

Epilepsy

Epileptic seizures are caused by electrical disturbances in the nerve cells in the brain. These seizures vary in their severity. Petit mal seizures are mild—the person will stare into space and may twitch slightly. Grand mal seizures are more extreme—the person will fall to the ground, become unconscious, and have convulsions. Most seizures begin in childhood; just one-fourth of new epileptics are adults. Epilepsy, which stems from erratic surges in the brain's electrical rhythms, affects almost 2.5 million people. Epilepsy can be caused by infection, meningitis, rickets, malnutrition, hypoglycemia, head injuries, fever, or allergies. Most of the time the specific cause is not discovered for each person.

Nutrition Issues

Long-term use of anticonvulsant medications is the most common treatment of epilepsy. As with any medication, the absorption of vitamins and minerals can be affected. Vitamins D, E, and B$_{12}$, and folic acid are the nutrients most likely to be affected by long-term use of seizure-prevention drugs.

A ketogenic diet (very high fat/low carbohydrate) is sometimes helpful in controlling seizures in children. Ketogenic diets are difficult to manage, and all foods eaten must be precisely weighed or measured. Most children are hospitalized for several days when the diet is started so they can be carefully monitored for side effects. Following the diet results in a metabolic condition called ketosis. Your body burns fat supplied from foods when there is not enough carbohydrate available for immediate energy needs. Ketones are what are leftover in your bloodstream after fat is metabolized. It's not known why ketone production can stop seizures in some children, because ketosis is a health hazard in almost every other instance. Growing children will not receive adequate amounts of many nutrients on this type of diet and supplementation is essential. According to Cindy Moore, M.S., R.D., F.A.D.A., of the Cleveland Clinic, "one-third of our pediatric patients with epilepsy become seizure free, one-third have a reduced number of seizures, and one-third see no change or improvement on a ketogenic diet."

The ketogenic diet was originally developed at Johns Hopkins and the Mayo Clinic in the 1920s for preventing seizures. When anticonvulsant medications were later developed, ketogenic diets lost popularity. A ketogenic diet should not be the first line of treatment for children with epilepsy. It's not a program to try on your own; close medical and nutritional supervision is required.

New Nutrition *Recommendations for Epilepsy*

- Choose a basic low-fat, nutrient-rich eating plan that includes plenty of fruits, vegetables, and whole grains (if not on a specialized ketogenic diet).
- Take a multivitamin and mineral supplement at 100 to 150 percent of the RDA for those not on the ketogenic diet and 150 to 300 percent of the RDA for children following the specialized eating plan.
- Do not attempt to try a ketogenic diet on your own. It can be dangerous if not closely planned and monitored.
- Avoid alcohol and caffeine since they can alter the action of anticonvulsant medications.

LINK UP to http://www.efa.org for the Epilepsy Foundation of America.

Fibromyalgia Syndrome

Twenty years ago fibromyalgia (fi-bro-my-AL-ja) was almost unheard of. Today, it's the second most commonly diagnosed musculoskeletal disorder and a hot area of research and debate. Pain is the most prominent symptom of fibromyalgia—a burning, gnawing ache that affects the soft tissues of your body. Muscles and the tendons that attach them to bone are the main targets of this disease. Perhaps the best way to tell the difference between arthritis and fibromyalgia is that arthritis causes joint deformity and fibromyalgia does not. Although many with fibromyalgia syndrome are aware of pain when they are resting, it is most noticeable when they use their muscles for repetitive activities. The presence and special pattern of "tender points" of muscle pain also separate fibromyalgia from other conditions. In addition to widespread pain, other common symptoms include a decreased sense of energy, disturbances of sleep, and varying degrees of anxiety and depression related to changed physical status.

Nutrition Issues

Because fibromyalgia often occurs in people with autoimmune diseases such as lupus and rheumatoid arthritis, some researchers think it, too, has an immune system basis. If that link proves true, then the same recommendations to increase antioxidant nutrients from foods would make sense.

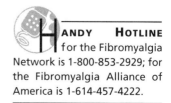

HANDY HOTLINE for the Fibromyalgia Network is 1-800-853-2929; for the Fibromyalgia Alliance of America is 1-614-457-4222.

Aerobic exercise, such as swimming and walking, improves muscle fitness and reduces muscle pain and tenderness. Heat and massage may also give short-term relief. Antidepressant medications may help elevate mood, improve quality of sleep, and relax muscles.

New Nutrition *Recommendations for Fibromyalgia*

- Choose a healthful diet. There is not enough information on potential links between fibromyalgia and diet to make any specific recommendations on food intake.
- Take a multivitamin and mineral supplement that provides 100 percent of the RDAs.

INK UP to http://www.fmnetnews.com for the Fibromyalgia Network.

Food Allergies, Sensitivities, and Intolerances

An allergic reaction occurs when your immune system mistakes a particular food as a harmful invader. Histamine (HISS-ta-meen) and other chemicals are launched to attack the food in a misguided effort to protect you from harm. This is the same system that responds to insect stings. The most common symptoms of an allergic reaction include hives, swelling (especially of the lips and face), difficult breathing (because of swelling in the throat or an asthmatic reaction), vomiting, diarrhea, cramping, and a drop in blood pressure. Allergic reactions are also called anaphylaxis (ann-uh-fah-LAX-iss) and can sometimes lead to death if not promptly treated. Anaphylaxis can be sudden or appear more like a slow-developing illness. Some noted allergists believe that repeated exposure to certain medicines or food ingredients can weaken the lining of your intestines. That makes it easier for allergens to pass through this barrier and come in direct contact with your immune system, provoking a reaction.

Nutrition Issues

The majority of adverse reactions to foods are not true food allergies, but rather are sensitivities or intolerances. The symptoms are similar, but these reactions—unlike allergies—either don't involve the immune system, or they involve a different part of the immune system than true allergies do.

Many people claim to be allergic to a food. But a true allergy is quite different from a food intolerance or sensitivity, which is what most people really have. Food intolerance is caused by the lack of enzymes needed for digestion, which results in food not being broken down properly. Undigested food can enter the bloodstream and cause a reaction. The symptoms are similar to those of food allergies. If you think you're allergic to whole groups of foods, have an evaluation by a board-certified allergist. Individuals most likely to have a real allergy to foods are those affected by nuts, legumes, and shellfish. Children have the highest rate of food allergies, but often outgrow them. On the other hand, allergies developed in adulthood are often with you for life.

In homes, schools, and institutions around the country people are eliminating certain foods from their diets, believing that allergic reactions to those foods are causing physical and emotional problems. Because you eat a variety of foods daily, it's easy to associate an unexplained symptom or discomfort with food. When you eliminate any food, you could be limiting your access to important vitamins and minerals.

The following food additives may cause adverse reactions in a few sensitive individuals: aspartame, benzoates, BHA, BHT, food colors, MSG, nitrates, parabens, and sulfites. Since there is no nutritional need for any of these substances, there is no harm in eliminating them. However, it will make food shopping much more difficult and time-consuming.

Sulfites are among the most widely used additives in prepared foods. Sulfiting agents are used to preserve foods and sanitize containers for certain beverages. When checking food labels, look for sulfur dioxide, sodium or potassium sulfite, bisulfite, and metabisulfite. Sulfites are commonly found in a variety of foods including bakery products, teas, 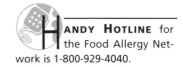ANDY **HOTLINE** for the Food Allergy Network is 1-800-929-4040.

ALLERGIC OR NOT?

To help distinguish among foods you just don't like, a food intolerance, and a true food allergy, ask yourself the following questions:

- After eating certain foods, do you break out into a rash or have itching or swelling?

- Do symptoms appear within minutes but not more than two hours after eating the food?

- Do you have a history of asthma or allergies to other things?

- Do allergies run in your family?

If you answered yes to most of these questions, then food allergy is more likely, as opposed to food intolerance. If you know that every time you eat a certain food you have a reaction, then it makes sense to avoid that food. If you aren't sure of the offending food, try an elimination diet under a doctor's or dietitian's supervision.

condiments, processed seafood, jams and jellies, dried fruit, fruit juices, frozen vegetables, soup mixes, beer, wine, and wine coolers.

Until recently, the highest levels of sulfites were in restaurant salad bars. However, because of the growing rate of reaction to sulfites, the Food and Drug Administration banned their use on fruits and vegetables intended to be served raw. The agency also mandated labeling for packaged foods that contain more than ten parts per million of any sulfiting agent, so that people

INK UP to http://www.foodallergy.org for the Food Allergy Network; it provides a wealth of resources and support group information.

sensitive to sulfites may easily identify products they should avoid.

A number of foods commonly believed to be allergenic are not. Chocolate, strawberries, tomatoes, citrus fruits, and corn are often blamed for allergic reactions, but they are rarely the cause. Sugar is not an allergenic food, although it is often thought to be.

GO FIGURE
Fewer than 2 percent of all adults suffer from true food allergies. Jordan Fink, M.D., chief allergist at the Medical College of Wisconsin and past president of the American Academy of Allergy and Immunology, agrees that "perhaps 5 percent of those individuals who think they have allergies will turn out to have one."

New Nutrition *Recommendations for Allergies*

- Check with a board-certified allergist to determine if you have a true allergy before you eliminate foods from your diet. Immune therapy or allergy shots have not been proven to work; neither has oral desensitization helped in eliminating food allergies. Bottom line: if you have a true food allergy, avoid the food.
- Take a calcium supplement with vitamin D that provides 100 percent of the RDA for these nutrients if you limit milk intake because of an allergy or intolerance.
- Always specify that you have a food allergy when eating at a restaurant. Ask how a food will be prepared and see that your waitperson checks with the chef to determine if any of the offending food is included in your selection. Never taste foods before asking questions.

INK UP to http://www.aaaai.org and the American Academy of Allergy, Asthma, and Immunology can help you locate a board-certified allergist in your area.

- Read food ingredient lists carefully when shopping at the supermarket. Become familiar with all the names used on labels; for example, sodium caseinate and casein are ingredients to avoid if you are allergic to milk protein. If you have questions about favorite foods, contact the manufacturers of the product.

LINK UP to http://www.foodallergy.org for more background information. Special allergy alerts and research studies from the Food Allergy Network.

Heart Disease

The most common first symptom of a heat attack may surprise you—it's death. That's right, sudden death is the first inkling that most people have signaling heart trouble. If you have chest pains, shortness of breath, or any of the other common symptoms, consider yourself fortunate. Heart disease is our nation's second most common cause of death among both men and women of all racial and ethnic groups. Three health-related behaviors—smoking, lack of enough exercise, and poor nutrition—are the major risk factors. At least 50 million Americans have some form of heart disease, including high blood pressure or high cholesterol. The American Heart Association estimates that the cost of heart disease in 1997 was $259 billion, including health care costs and lost productivity resulting from illness and death.

The Cholesterol Connection

Cholesterol is a building block of cells, vitamins, and hormones in the body. There is no dietary requirement for cholesterol from foods. Cholesterol is so essential that your liver manufactures all that you need. High blood cholesterol increases your risk for heart disease. Eating foods high in cholesterol is not the problem; other lifestyle factors contribute to the development of high blood cholesterol levels. Being overweight and inactive, eating too much total fat, and having too much saturated fat are the most significant reasons for elevated cholesterol levels (over 200 mg/dl). For every 1 percent reduction in total cholesterol, you can decrease your risk of heart disease by 2 percent. If your cholesterol is 240 mg/dl and you bring it down to 216 mg/dl, your risk decreases 20 percent. Some people have a rare genetic predisposition to high blood cholesterol that usually requires medication for effective cholesterol control.

Cholesterol is usually a fatlike substance present only in animal products such as meat, poultry, fish, milk and milk products, and egg yolks. Lower-fat foods do not contain less cholesterol than their full-fat versions. That's because cholesterol is found in almost every part of an animal or a human body.

Go **FIGURE** your cholesterol

High	240 or more
Borderline high	200–239
Desirable	below 200

Elevated cholesterol is a big risk factor for coronary heart disease. According to the land-mark Framingham study, which tracked cholesterol levels of five thousand men and women over twenty years, men with average blood cholesterol levels of 260 mg/dl had three times more heart attacks than men with average blood cholesterol levels of 195 mg/dl.

HDL (Good) and LDL (Bad) Cholesterol

Your total cholesterol level includes different types of cholesterol in your blood. Actually, your total cholesterol is not as important as the ratio between the good and bad forms. High-density lipoproteins (HDLs) are the good guys and low-density lipoproteins (LDLs) are the bad guys.

Your HDL level is a key factor in your risk of heart attack. For example, if your HDL level is low (below 35), you are at risk even if your total cholesterol is only 200. But if your HDL level is up (above 80), your risk is lower—even with total cholesterol as high as 240. The higher the HDL, the better.

Go **FIGURE** your HDL level

Low	below 35
Borderline low	35–39
Desirable	60 or more

LDL cholesterol is the bad stuff that clogs your arteries. You want low levels of the low-density lipoproteins. LDLs can be small or large; small LDLs have recently been linked to undesirable low levels of HDL (good) cholesterol and to high levels of triglycerides. One in three men and one in six postmenopausal women have more small LDLs than large ones and may therefore be at higher risk for coronary heart disease.

Go **FIGURE** your LDL level

High	160 or above
Borderline high	130–159
Desirable	below 130
Desirable for people with heart disease	below 100

Triglycerides

Triglycerides are fats found in the bloodstream. If your triglyc-erides are high, you can actually see white fatty streaks in a sample of blood being drawn. Most

Go **FIGURE** your triglyceride level

Very High	1,000 or more
High	400–1,000
Borderline high	200–399
Desirable	below 200

people with elevated triglycerides either have a genetic link or consume excessive amounts of alcohol.

Lp (a)

Lp (a) (el-PEE, lit-tull a) is a form of LDL "bad" cholesterol. It is emerging as another risk factor for heart disease. An elevated level of Lp (a) in your blood is a concern. However, it is not clear how to lower a high Lp (a) level. Some preliminary findings point to aspirin, red wine, and omega-3 fatty acids from fish as possibly lowering Lp (a) levels. More research is needed before specific dietary recommendations can be made, but following a heart-healthy diet is a good start.

Nutrition Issues

Diets to prevent heart disease always begin with what you can't have or must limit. Try a new approach. Eat more fruits and vegetables, add in a variety of whole-grain breads and cereals, seek out lean meats, poultry, plenty of fish, and skim or low-fat dairy products. Choose foods as close to how they were grown as possible.

L INK UP to http://www.nhlbi.nih.gov or http://www.americanheart.org for more specifics on the step diets if you have heart disease and need guidance on this plan.

These are the most popular eating plans to prevent or reverse heart disease.

Step I Diet. Designed by the National Cholesterol Education Program as the first step in treating high blood cholesterol. This low-fat plan (30 percent of total calories) restricts saturated fat (8 to 10 percent of total calories) and dietary cholesterol (less than 300 mg), and provides enough calories to achieve or maintain a healthy weight. If blood cholesterol levels aren't lowered in three to six months, the Step II Diet should be tried.

Step II Diet. A more restrictive version of the Step I diet. Saturated fat is kept to less than 7 percent of total calories, and dietary cholesterol is held at 200 mg. If these dietary changes don't result in lower blood cholesterol, then medications may be prescribed.

Pritikin Diet. Created by Nathan Pritikin in the late 1950s, this severely low–fat diet (5 to 10 percent of total calories from fat) focuses on grain, fruits, and vegetables. Such significant fat restrictions are not for everyone. However, if you're highly motivated to lower your cholesterol, it can have good results.

Ornish Diet. In the late 1970s, Dr. Dean Ornish developed a very low–fat diet (less than 10 percent of total calories from fat), which he claims can even reverse severe heart disease without drugs or surgery. As with the Pritikin Diet, many people find the severe fat limitations a challenge to stick with.

 LINK UP to http://www.allhealth.com/ornish/articles/gen/0,4260,6754_125 300,00.html for key elements of the Ornish diet from iVillage's allHealth site.

Generally speaking, there's plenty of evidence that antioxidants may prevent clogging of the arteries by blocking the oxidation of LDL. Vitamins E and C are showing great promise, and dietary beta-carotene has also shown positive effects. Studies show mixed results on garlic supplements, but including plenty of fresh garlic may help.

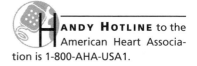 **H**ANDY **HOTLINE** to the American Heart Association is 1-800-AHA-USA1.

New Nutrition *Recommendations for Avoiding Heart Disease*

- Choose an eating plan that will work for you and stay with it for life.
- Maintain a healthy weight through sensible eating and regular physical activity.
- Take a multivitamin and mineral supplement with 100 percent of the RDA. Extra B6 and folic acid may help if you have elevated homocysteine levels, unless discouraged by your doctor.
- Consider taking fish oil supplements. They may have the potential for lowering the risk for blocked blood vessels and heart attacks, but their current effectiveness and proper dosage haven't been determined.
- Don't take coenzyme Q-10 even though it has potential as an antioxidant and could protect against heart disease. Because research into coenzyme Q-10 is still at a relatively early stage, the use of supplements isn't advisable.

 LINK UP to http://www.americanheart.org for the American Heart Association.

High Blood Pressure

High blood pressure, or hypertension, affects nearly 60 million Americans, or one in four adults. Historically, treatment has alternated between an emphasis on diet and use of antihypertensive drugs. The use of drugs

WHAT YOUR DOCTOR DOESN'T KNOW

A 1998 survey to determine physicians' nutrition knowledge about diet and high blood fats showed that many doctors have a lot to learn. This study, reported in the journal *Circulation*, found that of the doctors who responded:

- 82 percent did not know that a low-fat diet would decrease HDL levels. (It does.)

- 70 percent thought a low-fat diet had no more than 20 percent of calories from fat. (It's 30 percent or less.)

- 40 percent incorrectly believed that dietary fat raises blood triglyceride levels. (It doesn't.)

- 30 percent didn't identify olive oil as a monounsaturated fat. (It is.)

This is another reason to ask your doctor for a referral to a qualified dietitian. It's clear that the National Cholesterol Education Program needs to change their recommendation that diet counseling by physicians be the first treatment for management of high levels of cholesterol and blood fats.

should never be the first option because of potential serious side effects. The nondrug approach is far safer and more effective. Blood pressure is considered to be elevated when readings are above 140/90. The upper number is called the systolic pressure, which is the pressure that occurs when the heart contracts and pushes blood out to the body. The bottom number is called the diastolic pressure. This is the pressure in the arteries when the heart relaxes between beats.

High blood pressure is a significant risk factor for developing heart disease. Not only does hypertension increase the risk of heart attacks, but it also increases the risk of stroke and kidney disease. Of the 60 million people with hypertension, almost half are women. A 1998 study from the National Institutes of Health indicates that uncontrolled high blood pressure increases loss of brain cells associated with aging. Fewer brain cells mean your memory won't be as good and your thinking patterns will be fuzzier.

Nutrition Issues
Only about 10 percent of Americans with high blood pressure can lower blood pressure significantly with a low-sodium diet. Eating lots of fruits, vegetables, and skim or low-fat dairy products is more beneficial than

cutting back on salt for most people trying to get their blood pressure in control. Potassium, calcium, and magnesium from these foods are thought to be key to blood pressure improvements. A modest weight loss of just ten pounds,

HANDY HOTLINE for the National Heart, Lung, and Blood Institute is 1-800-575-9355.

especially if you have lots of tummy fat, can often reduce elevated blood pressure to normal levels.

Coenzyme Q-10 may improve hypertension, producing a decline in both systolic and diastolic blood pressure, but use of this supplement should be managed by your health care provider. Garlic has lowered blood pressure in some studies. Eating just one clove of garlic per day in foods may have some blood pressure–lowering benefits. Do not take any form of licorice. Even relatively small amounts (50 grams or less) of licorice can raise blood pressure.

Regular use of nonsteroidal anti-inflammatory drugs (NSAIDs) may raise blood pressure, particularly in older people. They may also impair the action of beta-blocking medicines that lower blood pressure. NSAIDs include ibuprofen (Advil, Motrin) and naproxen (Aleve).

LINK UP to http://www.nhlbi.nih.gov for the National Heart, Lung, and Blood Institute.

Selected Studies

Several observational studies of high blood pressure and produce consumption have indicated that fruits and vegetables may help lower blood pressure. A carefully controlled clinical trial has confirmed this. The trial, called Dietary Approaches to Stop Hypertension (DASH), involved randomly assigning 133 people with hypertension to spend two months on one of three diets: a regimen rich in both produce and lean dairy products, rich in produce but low in dairy products, or low in both produce and dairy. The combination of a high-produce, high-dairy diet reduced blood pressure readings significantly compared with a low-produce, low-dairy diet. Fruits and vegetables accounted for a large portion of the pressure reductions (*New England Journal of Medicine*, 1997). Widespread adoption of the DASH diet is estimated to be able to reduce heart disease by 15 percent and stroke by 27 percent.

New Nutrition *Recommendations for High Blood Pressure*

- Try the DASH diet. Eat eight to ten servings of fruits and vegetables each day, two to three servings of low-fat dairy foods, seven to eight servings of grains, and up to two serving of lean meat daily. Also included are four to five servings of nuts, seeds, and beans each week.
- Maintain a healthy weight. The benefits of weight loss can't be

overemphasized. Overweight adults are 50 percent more likely than normal-weight adults to have hypertension.

- Drink less alcohol. Drinking three or more alcoholic beverages a day can raise blood pressure.
- Get regular exercise. It will help keep both your weight and your blood pressure low.
- Make peace with your salt intake. If eating less salt and less foods high in sodium helps lower your blood pressure, then stay on a low-sodium diet. If you are used to lower-sodium foods, don't start eating more. Foods rich in potassium, calcium, and magnesium may help blunt the effects of sodium on your blood pressure.

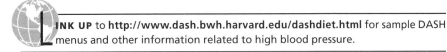

LINK UP to http://www.dash.bwh.harvard.edu/dashdiet.html for sample DASH menus and other information related to high blood pressure.

HIV/AIDS

Acquired immunodeficiency syndrome (AIDS) is a viral infection that causes a harmful antibody response in your immune system. The HIV (human immunodeficiency virus) gene actually gets into your cells and multiplies. As the HIV spreads, it weakens your immune system so that you are unable to fight off many normal infections. In a healthy immune system, the white blood cells surround a virus and destroy it. With AIDS, the HIV virus is surrounded but the white cells can't kill it, and the virus reproduces unchecked.

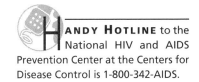

HANDY **HOTLINE** to the National HIV and AIDS Prevention Center at the Centers for Disease Control is 1-800-342-AIDS.

Nutrition Issues

It can take two to five years (or longer) after the initial infection for symptoms of the AIDS virus to appear. When the virus becomes more active, early symptoms are vague and include weight loss, fatigue, diarrhea, headaches, swollen glands, fever, and loss of appetite. A common symptom is thrush (white patches in the mouth), which indicates a suppressed immune system. When these symptoms occur, they are the signs that the body has been depleted of many nutrients and may develop full-blown deficiencies. Many trace elements such as zinc and selenium are used up before you even notice any symptoms.

Diet is an important part of the battle against HIV infection. In general, a nutritious variety of foods provides the best combination of nutrients. What you eat is especially important when taking drug therapy for HIV infection. In many instances it makes the difference between success and failure of your medications. In order for medications to get into the body, they must be absorbed by the gastrointestinal tract (through the stomach and intestines). Some drugs require stomach acid (with no food in the stomach) to be absorbed while others need to be absorbed in the presence of food. The guidance of a dietitian in meal planning and spacing can also help alleviate some drug side effects.

Malnutrition is a very serious problem for people with AIDS. Life expectancy is directly related to how much body mass you can keep. A loss of 55 percent of lean muscle weight is practically a death sentence to those with AIDS. Another source of malnutrition comes from ongoing infections, which change how all nutrients are metabolized.

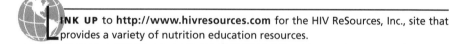

INK UP to http://www.hivresources.com for the HIV ReSources, Inc., site that provides a variety of nutrition education resources.

Food safety is as critical as good nutrition in the management of AIDS. Suppressed immunity dramatically increases the risk of food-borne illness and the severity of complications. There are bacteria and germs lurking in almost everything we eat and drink. When levels of these contaminants get high enough, they can make you sick. It takes far less contamination to make you ill when you have AIDS. See Chapter 3 and the appendices for a complete look at necessary food safety precautions.

INK UP to http://www.cdc.gov for the Centers for Disease Control information on HIV/AIDS data and research.

New Nutrition *Recommendations for HIV/AIDS*

- Consult a registered dietitian (RD) as soon as you are diagnosed for a complete nutritional assessment including weight, height, body fat, lean muscle mass, and BMI. Your RD should also explain your lab results from blood and urine samples. Keep as much lean body mass as possible by staying active and eating a variety of foods.
- Focus on maintaining your weight. Eating small, frequent meals can help to increase the number of calories you eat.
- Eat plenty of quality protein and antioxidant-rich fruits, vegetables, and grains to keep your immune system strong.
- Wash all fruits and vegetables with a nonsoap-based produce rinse (such as Fit®) to avoid food-borne infections.
- Never eat raw or undercooked eggs or soft ripe cheeses. Be sure ground meats are cooked well done. Use a food thermometer to check temperatures.

- Drink bottled water if your local water supply doesn't meet federal safety standards. (See Chapter 2 for how to check your local water quality.)
- Use bleach or an antibacterial solution (1 tablespoon to 1 gallon water) to wipe kitchen surfaces.
- Take a multivitamin/mineral supplement that provides 100 percent of the RDAs.
- Check with your health care provider if you are on antifolate drug treatment; you may need extra folic acid.
- Try to decrease caffeine to help prevent stomach irritation.
- Take additional supplements of vitamins A, D, E, and K if you develop steatorrhea (fatty diarrhea).

LINK UP to http://www.noah.cuny.edu/aids/aids.html for many up-to-date resources on AIDS and nutrition from the New York Online Access to Health (NOAH).

Inflammatory Bowel Disease

Crohn's disease and colitis are types of inflammatory bowel diseases (IBDs). They are chronic diseases without a known cause or cure. An estimated 2 million Americans have been diagnosed with IBDs.

Colitis is an inflammation of the inner lining of the digestive tract affecting the colon or the rectum. Crohn's disease is an inflammation of all the layers of the digestive tract affecting any part from the mouth to the anus. It's because the symptoms and complications are similar that they both are grouped under the heading of IBDs. Common symptoms include weight loss, fever, abdominal pain, and diarrhea.

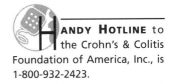

HANDY HOTLINE to the Crohn's & Colitis Foundation of America, Inc., is 1-800-932-2423.

Nutrition Issues

Malnutrition is a significant problem in IBDs for several reasons. First, it's pretty miserable to live in chronic pain, and that lowers the desire to eat. Second, scar tissue forms along the digestive tract as a result of inflammation. This scarring interferes with normal absorption of nutrients and decreases the available supply of nutrients and energy. This is especially important in children because high levels of calories and nutrients are essential for optimal growth.

Sometimes it's necessary to rely on liquid meal replacement supplements to provide enough calories and nutrients during severe bouts of symptoms. Ideally these supplements are aids to a wholesome diet and not used in place of eating real foods. Extra supplements are not typically recommended and may even cause more harm, such as an increase in diarrhea. IBD is one of the few conditions that benefits from a lower fiber intake. Too much roughage can irritate an already sensitive digestive tract.

New Nutrition *Recommendations for IBD*

- Individualize your optimal nutrition plan if you have IBD. What may work for one person may not work so well for another person.
- Choose foods that are rich in nutrients whenever possible. You may need to avoid some higher-fiber foods if they cause pain or complications of your symptoms.
- Spread meals out over the course of the day. Five small meals instead of three large ones may help decrease side effects.
- Eliminate a particular food for several weeks if it seems to intensify your symptoms. Then slowly reintroduce it to see if it has any effect.
- Avoid supplemental vitamins and minerals unless they have been specifically prescribed by your gastroenterologist.
- Try substituting a liquid diet meal (Carnation Instant Breakfast, Ensure, or Boost) to provide calories and a source of nutrients when you can't eat.
- Be cautious in your consumption of herbal teas. Tannins and other compounds may irritate your digestive system.

INK UP to http://www.ccfa.org for the Crohn's & Colitis Foundation of America, Inc.

Macular Degeneration

Macular degeneration is the deterioration and functional loss of the yellow spot on the retina, which is responsible for central vision. The more the yellow spot deteriorates, the more vision is lost. Lutein is a yellow pigment in the human eye (it also gives marigolds their golden yellow color). Zeaxanthin is another bright yellow pigment that is almost identical in structure to lutein. Together lutein and zeaxanthin are the pigments that color the tiny spot on your eye yellow. The density of yellow color is proportional to the amount of lutein and zeaxanthin it contains. Macular density gets worse as macular degeneration progresses because of the loss of these pigments.

Macular degeneration is a leading cause of blindness in people over 55 years old. It can strike anyone and works slowly and silently to destroy vision. Medical research studies show

ANDY HOTLINE to the Lighthouse National Center for Vision and Aging is 1-800-334-5497.

that as many as one-fourth of all people over the age of 65 have a measurable level of macular degeneration, and there is no treatment for the disease at present. The good news is that macular degeneration can sometimes be prevented or the progressive loss of sight slowed.

Nutrition Issues

It may be possible to reverse the process of macular degeneration somewhat by nutritional intervention. Eating more dark green leafy vegetables such as collards and spinach will add extra carotenoids, lutein, and zeaxanthin. Too much saturated fat may increase the risk of age-related macular degeneration.

Selected Studies

A team of medical researchers from Erasmus University Medical School in Rotterdam found that macular degeneration is much more common and severe in people who have close relatives with the condition. They suspect that up to 25 percent of macular degeneration cases may be genetically determined (*Archives of Ophthalmology*, December 1998). However, it isn't clear whether there is one gene causing the problem, several genes, or if there is some combination of genes that make family members susceptible.

New Nutrition *Recommendations for Macular Degeneration*

- Eat at least one or two servings daily of a dark green leafy vegetable such as spinach, kale, or collard greens. These vegetables supply a high amount of lutein and zeaxanthin, the yellow carotenoid pigments absolutely necessary for the health of the macula.
- Eat a serving of blueberries every day. Blueberries are especially high in total antioxidative activity. Fresh or frozen blueberries are equally good choices.
- Try bilberry extract if you don't like blueberries (it ranks even higher than blueberries for antioxidant capacity). However, eating whole fruit (blueberry or bilberry) may offer other beneficial substances, which may not be present in the extract.
- Eat a total of at least five servings per day of vegetables or fruits to increase the total antioxidant activity of the blood.
- Get an adequate zinc intake of 15 mg per day. This amount of zinc is readily supplied by any good multivitamin and mineral tablet.
- Take antioxidant supplements to equal 400 IU per day of all-natural vitamin E consisting of mixed tocopherols and a supplement of 250 mg per day of vitamin C. Be sure to add up the amounts in your multivitamin and mineral supplements before choosing individual products.
- Drink one glass of red or purple grape juice or red wine every day for its protective antioxidant activity.

- Do not take ginkgo biloba extract. Although it is an excellent antioxidant, its consumption carries a very small risk of hemorrhage in the brain, usually a lethal condition. It is doubtful whether any potential benefit outweighs the risk, no matter how small.

INK UP to http://www.eyesight.org or http://www.eyenet.org for the American Academy of Ophthalmology Eyenet.

Menopause

Menopause, also referred to as "the change of life," is the point at which women stop ovulating. Menopause affects each woman differently. For most women, menstrual cycles become less regular at about age 50. The cycles eventually cease. Menopause is caused when the ovaries lose their ability to release hormones. The menopausal phase can last up to five years. Although estrogen levels drop during the postmenopausal period, the hormone does not entirely disappear.

Typical menopausal symptoms include hot flashes, dizziness, headache, shortness of breath, and depression. These are thought to be the result of fluctuating estrogen levels. To help control symptoms, a small amount of estrogen daily will help. Check with your doctor about the benefits and risks of hormone replacement therapy.

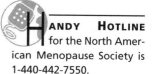

ANDY HOTLINE for the North American Menopause Society is 1-440-442-7550.

Nutrition Issues

Many women complain that weight gain speeds up during menopause. The slightest fluctuation in estrogen and progesterone affects metabolism and appetite. Weight gain seems to be the body's response to this major reorganization of the female hormone system. In addition, increased calorie intake due to the stresses of coping with such profound body changes may also contribute to weight gain.

The abrupt loss of female hormones during menopause leads to a decrease in calcium absorption and increases the rate of bone loss. It's essential to compensate for these losses through extra servings of dairy products or calcium supplementation. Anyone who takes in high levels of calcium (over 1,000 mg/day) should aim for at least 400 mg of magnesium to keep these essential nutrients in a balanced ratio of 2:1.

Soy and flax, plants rich in estrogenlike compounds, have been heavily promoted as helping to ease the variety of symptoms that occur with the change of life. Studies have shown that fewer than a quarter of Japanese menopausal women, whose normal diet contains lots of soy protein, complain of hot flashes. However, these findings have been questioned by some who say that the Japanese culture may discourage women from complaining about symptoms even if they do experience them.

Less iron is required for menopausal women because they no longer have monthly blood losses. It's still important to choose high-iron foods, since most women eat so few calories.

Herbs have long been used to help control the symptoms of menopause. Ginseng may lessen the intensity of hot flashes and other symptoms, but too much can have powerful effects on the female reproductive system and may cause uterine bleeding. (For those not yet menopausal, evening primrose oil may help alleviate premenstrual symptoms.)

Selected Studies

Researchers in Italy studied 104 women (not on hormone replacement therapy) who were really sweating out menopause, having at least seven moderate to severe hot flashes a day. Half of the women were given soy protein, half a placebo. By the end of the twelfth week, the number of hot flashes per day dropped by nearly half in the women taking soy (*Obstetrics & Gynecology*, January 1998). Women taking the placebo also had a reduction in hot flashes, but only by about a third. The soy didn't seem to help with other menopausal symptoms, such as headaches or insomnia. The Italian researchers had a tough time getting volunteers to stick with the study, because the soy powder used wasn't very appealing.

New Nutrition *Recommendations for Menopause*

- Maintain a healthy weight by increasing regular physical activity. Calorie needs decrease as your age increases. Since most women eat a minimal amount of calories to begin with, burning more calories is the best solution for preventing undesirable weight gain.
- Choose foods rich in calcium and magnesium to curb bone loss. If you can't or won't consume dairy products, choose a calcium carbonate or calcium citrate supplement.
- Experiment with foods like soy and flax or supplements of ginseng or evening primrose oil to determine if they help reduce menopausal symptoms. Choose only one supplement at a time so that you can effectively judge its impact.

INK UP to http://www.menopause.org for the North American Menopause Society.

Migraines and Headaches

It starts as a hot pain behind your eye and builds to a peak until you can't stand light, noise, or even the slightest touch. You just want to lie in dark silence. Migraines are a whole dimension beyond headaches. Migraines tend to begin in your head, but as they progress they can wreak havoc on your whole body with severe head throbbing, nausea, vomiting, dizziness, cold hands, tremors, and sensitivity to light and sound.

Migraines are thought to be triggered by an electrical spasm in the back of the brain. The spasm causes blood vessels in this area to constrict, while the vessels at the top of the brain dilate. Blood goes into the arteries around your temples, causing throbbing pain and inflammation in the brain covering. Migraines can be temporary or last a day or two. The serotonin level may play a large role in the triggering of the spasm.

HANDY HOTLINE to the National Headache Foundation is 1-888-643-5552.

Migraines are largely hereditary, and women tend to develop them three times more often than men. Nearly 18 million Americans suffer migraines, and more than 157 million workdays are lost each year because of them, according to the National Headache Foundation in Chicago.

Nutrition Issues

Many things can bring on an attack of migraine: changing hormone levels prior to menstruation or during ovulation, poor eating or sleeping habits, stress, chemicals in food (including additives and preservatives), or low blood sugar.

NSAIDs (nonsteroidal anti-inflammatory drugs such as aspirin, ibuprofen, and naproxen) often cause side effects, especially upset stomachs. These pain medications are called simple analgesics because they contain a single ingredient, in contrast to combined analgesics, which contain additional ingredients such as caffeine.

Magnesium may play a role in preventing or reducing the frequency of migraine headaches. Rich food sources of magnesium include cocoa, chocolate, most nuts, fish and shellfish, legumes, kelp, corn, soybean sprouts, lima beans, whole-wheat muffins, taco shells, bran flakes, toasted wheat germ, brown rice, grain and grain products, dried figs, dried pears, bananas, and dark green leafy vegetables. Feverfew is an herb that may also provide some relief for migraines.

Probably the best news for migraine sufferers is that chocolate has been taken off the list of foods that may trigger these severe headaches. Phenols in red wine and tyramine in aged cheese can increase a hormone release that constricts blood vessels. When the vessels suddenly rebound to open, a throbbing sensation results. Caffeine can temporarily prevent a headache by dilating blood vessels, but too much will cause overdilation and that can be as painful as constriction. Some people are so sensitive to caffeine that even a little will cause a headache. Others get headaches from caffeine overconsumption. Food additives, including those containing sulfites, may cause headaches in some individuals. Another source of headaches is hunger.

Selected Studies

A scientific review of feverfew studies showed that this herb tended to be more effective than a placebo in the prevention of migraine headaches (*Cephalalgia*, December 1998). The power of the placebo was fairly effective at prevention. Since there are few risks associated with feverfew, you may want to give it a try for four to six weeks.

New Nutrition *Recommendations for Migraines and Headaches*

- Avoid foods that seem to trigger a reaction; common triggers include red wine (phenols) and aged cheese (tyramine). There is no particular way of eating that universally impacts the occurrence of migraine headaches.
- Include plenty of food sources of magnesium or consider a supplement if you can't regularly eat these foods.
- Eat small, more frequent meals to help prevent hunger, which can also be a headache trigger.

LINK UP to http://www.migrainehelp.com for more resources and information.

Obesity

If you weigh 20 percent or more above your healthy weight, you're obese (carrying an excess accumulation of fat). Being overweight is defined as excess body weight that includes muscle, bone, fat, and water. It is possible that you may be overweight, but not obese, if you're physically fit and have lots of heavy, dense muscle mass.

Obesity is an important and dangerous disease. Despite the abundance of low-calorie and fat-free foods, Americans are getting fatter. Did you know that obesity is considered a risk factor for half of the ten leading causes of death in the United States? Carrying around an excess of body fat increases a person's risk for developing many potentially fatal diseases, including coronary heart disease, stroke, hypertension, diabetes, and some types of cancer.

Nutrition Issues

Name any diet and someone's probably lost weight on it. Losing weight is relatively simple; it's keeping those extra pounds off that's difficult. Remember, diets don't work permanently. It's attitudes and lifestyle changes that determine if the pounds you shed will stay off. A sedentary lifestyle is the single most critical factor in the explosion of obesity worldwide.

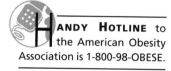

HANDY **HOTLINE** to the American Obesity Association is 1-800-98-OBESE.

Diet Program Pitfalls

Americans spend over $30 billion a year on diet programs and products in an attempt to lose weight. Unfortunately, most will fail. Here's a look at the pitfalls of popular diet programs.

Diet Method	Premise	Why It Fails	Potential Side Effects
Fasting (no solid foods for one or more days)	Quick weight loss, natural process that detoxifies your system.	Weight loss is from water, not fat. Can't be maintained over the long run. Difficult to stop eating and be able to work or be socially active.	Repeated fasting may actually decrease your metabolism, making it harder to lose weight permanently. Fasting stresses your body systems.
Liquid meal replacements (canned shakes or drinks)	Control calorie intake by replacing one or more meals with special beverage.	Not a satisfying replacement for food. No change in eating or exercise behaviors.	Doesn't promote a healthful lifestyle. Overuse may cause nutrient deficiencies.
Over-the-counter pills (variety of appetite suppressants, bulking agents)	Decreases your appetite so you feel like eating less. Usually contain phenylpropanol amine (PPA) and/or caffeine.	PPA has been repeatedly proven ineffective in controlling appetite or weight.	Caffeine may cause elevated blood pressure, irritability. Over time one may need stronger doses and develop a dependency.
Prepackaged meals (ready-to-eat meals packaged and sold by weight-loss programs or companies)	You don't have to think about choosing foods or practice portion control.	It's not reasonable to eat prepackaged meals as a lifetime weight-control method. Alienates family and friends. Often quite expensive.	Lack of variety can lead to nutritional deficiencies. Most prepackaged meals are low in fiber and don't include enough fruits, vegetables, and whole grains.

Diet Method	Premise	Why It Fails	Potential Side Effects
Surgery (stomach stapling, gastric bypass)	Quick, dramatic weight loss without dieting or exercise.	Doesn't promote change in behaviors needed to keep weight off. Most people regain weight.	Obese people are at much higher risk for surgical complications, including death. Chronic diarrhea and malabsorption are permanent side effects of these surgeries and often cause malnutrition.
Very low-calorie diets (under 1,000 calories)	Quick weight loss due to dramatic calorie reduction.	Most people can't keep calories this low without feeling deprived. May binge eat to compensate.	Your body can adjust to needing fewer calories by lowering your metabolism. May lead to eating disorders.
High-protein, low-carbohydrate diets	Quick weight loss, able to eat lots of meat and fat.	People get bored quickly. You may feel nauseated after 4 to 5 days. Not a healthful long-term eating plan.	Constipation, dehydration, and bad breath are noticeable. This diet lacks disease-fighting nutrients and fiber.

New Nutrition *Recommendations to Avoid Obesity*

- Get regular exercise; at least thirty minutes a day of activity equivalent to brisk walking is recommended. You don't have to do it all at once; three shorter periods of ten minutes each are just as effective.
- Monitor what you eat. Focus on healthful eating, not deprivation diets. Choose foods that enhance your health such as fruits, vegetables, whole grains, lean meats, and low-fat dairy products. Seek foods for their nutrient benefits, not their calorie content.
- Lose weight slowly; losing one pound per week is considered most effective. If you are overweight, losing as little as 5 to 10 percent of your body weight can improve your health.

Selected Studies

A study of 861 women (20 to 45 years old) completed at the University of Minnesota now proves a correlation among fast-food consumption, television viewing, and increased obesity in the United States. Researchers found that the women who watched television ate more fast-food meals than non-TV watchers. This relationship was strongest in low-income women (*American Journal of Public Health,* February 1998). This study suggests that abundance of fast-food and excessive television viewing can contribute to obesity. It's the same old message—be more active, and eat more fruits and vegetables.

Older women don't burn off the fat in large meals as well as younger women, concluded a study from the Jean Mayer USDA Human Nutrition Research Center on Aging at Tufts University. When fed a meal of 1,000 calories, women in their 80s burned fewer calories and stored more fat than women in their 20s. Meals with 250 to 500 calories were metabolized the same in both groups (*American Journal of Clinical Nutrition,* vol. 66, 1997). If you're getting up in years, it makes sense to limit how often you eat calorie-laden meals.

 INK UP to http://www.obesity.org for the American Obesity Association.

Osteoporosis

Osteoporosis (meaning "porous bones") is a bone-thinning disease affecting one out of every three postmenopausal women, and elderly men, too. Symptomless throughout most of life, osteoporosis usually first reveals itself as a hip or spine fracture in old age. While there is no cure for osteoporosis, its debilitating effect can be prevented.

Robert Heaney, M.D., one of the leading U.S. calcium researchers, says, "Osteoporosis is an adolescent concern that doesn't express itself until old age." Osteoporosis affects 25 million people in the United States, causes 1.5 million bone fractures a year, and costs $10 billion annually in medical costs. There is no doubt that the best protection against future bone loss is to build the best skeleton possible during the growth years of 9 to 19.

Bone is a living tissue, just like skin or muscle. In fact, 20 percent of bone tissue is replaced every year through the process called bone remodeling. Bone-eating cells called osteoclasts break down bone, creating holes; then bone-building cells called osteoblasts come along and fill up those holes with fresh new bone. The whole process can take four to six months.

Here are the main reasons that women, especially older women, are at such high risk:

- Women have less bone mass at adulthood than men do because of their typically smaller frame size. As women age, they are therefore more vulnerable to any loss of bone.
- The male hormone testosterone protects men's bones as they age into their 60s and 70s. Women, on the other hand, need the hormone estrogen for bone health and density; after menopause, estrogen levels fall.

- Younger women who have anorexia and athletes with amenorrhea also may be at risk for bone mass loss due to decreased estrogen.
- Women typically consume less calcium-rich foods than men.

Nutrition Issues

Calcium helps in the bone-building process by contributing to increased bone density and strength. Infants have far more bone-building osteoblasts at work than bone-eating osteoclasts. That's why their milk-based diet is perfectly suited to provide so much calcium and vitamin D. During adolescence, bone development really shifts into high gear. Nearly half of all bone is formed during the teen years. This is a time when calcium is crucial to build strong bones. Unfortunately, it is also a time when teens start replacing milk with soft drinks.

By the early 20s, you are still in the prime bone-building years. Even though the length of your bones is set, they can still grow in density and strength. Bone growth through your early 30s creates a reserve supply for the future. The peak bone mass that you reach in your early 30s is the maximum amount of bone you will ever have. As you age, you will be using up bone and calcium faster than you can replace it. Between the ages of 35 and 45, you begin to use up calcium faster than ever before. Exercise and continued intake of calcium are critical for maintaining bone density. By age 45, you need to protect against a net loss of bone, which occurs when you are losing more bone material than you are making.

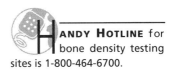

ANDY HOTLINE for bone density testing sites is 1-800-464-6700.

In the United States, the recommendations for daily calcium intake are twice as high as in other countries because Americans have greater urinary losses of calcium. There are two theories that suggest why this happens. Typical American diets have a high ratio of phosphorus to calcium, about 5:1; the ideal ratio is 1:1. High levels of phosphorus reduce calcium absorption, contributing to slow, continuous demineralization of bone tissue. Most soft drinks, particularly diet versions, are high in phosphorus, further upsetting the body's balance of phosphorus and calcium. American diets also tend to be high in protein, and you lose extra calcium through urination with high-protein diets. That's because protein foods are high in phosphorus and low in calcium, adding to the imbalance.

Calcium absorption is blocked if you drink more than two alcoholic drinks a day. The caffeine in coffee, tea, and soda (at levels of about ten cups a day) also interferes with calcium absorption.

Food plans that limit dairy products and are high in protein can deplete the bones of calcium. Vegetarians who avoid milk products may be at risk unless they are careful to get enough calcium. Crash diets or fasting also contributes to accumulated bone loss.

Those with inadequate amounts of the digestive enzyme lactase may develop lactose intolerance, a condition that makes it difficult to ingest milk products without discomfort. This can result in calcium deficiencies in people who avoid dairy foods because they cannot tolerate them comfortably. Fortunately, lactose-reduced milk and dairy products are now available, as are lactase tablets (e.g., Lactaid and Dairy Ease) that can be taken with dairy products.

Too much sodium increases urinary calcium loss. If you consume a modest amount of sodium (2,000 to 3,000 mg/day), you need about 1,200 mg of calcium. If your sodium intake is higher, you probably need more calcium.

Vitamin D enables the absorption of calcium. The natural way to get vitamin D is through sun exposure (see vitamin D in Chapter 5). Otherwise, you need about 400 IU of vitamin D a day from fortified foods or supplements. Milk is fortified with vitamin D to guard against this problem.

Bone health is perhaps the only health issue where being overweight or obese most of your life is a positive factor. The heavier you are, the more stress you place on your bones, and that's a good thing. Weight-bearing exercise strengthens bone tissue. Of course, it's better for your overall health to have that extra weight be in the form of dumbbells, not fat deposits on your body.

Selected Studies

- Seven- to 9-year-old children who drank an extra ⅔ cup of milk every school day for two years had higher bone density fourteen years later than children who did not have additional milk (*American Journal of Clinical Nutrition,* September 1992). Encourage children to choose milk for most meals and snacks.

- Twelve-year-old girls who increase their calcium intake from 900 mg per day to 1,200 mg daily for eighteen months had a higher total body and spine bone density than girls who did not eat the additional calcium (*Journal of the American Medical Association,* August 1993). You can get an extra 300 mg of calcium in 1 glass of skim milk or 1 cup of low-fat yogurt. The girls who ate the extra calcium-rich foods did not gain weight compared to other girls in the study.

- Supplementation with 400 mg of calcium citrate two times a day can decrease bone loss and stabilize bone density in the spine, hip, and arms of postmenopausal women (presentation at the joint meeting of the American Society for Bone and Mineral Research and the International Bone and Mineral Society, December 1998). It appears that the citrate form of calcium is better absorbed on an empty stomach than other common forms of calcium.

HANDY **HOTLINE** for the National Dairy Council is 1-800-426-8271, and the American Dietetic Association Nutrition Hot Line is 1-800-366-1655; both organizations can provide a wealth of information on calcium sources and osteoporosis prevention.

New Nutrition *Recommendations for Osteoporosis*

- Build the best skeleton possible during the growth years; it's the best protection against future bone problems. Eat at least 1,000 to 1,500 milligrams of calcium per day from foods.
- Consume three calcium-rich dairy foods a day, along with generous amounts of green leafy vegetables. Choose nondairy foods that have been fortified with extra calcium, such as orange juice and rice.
- Use calcium supplements if you need them to assist in meeting your calcium needs.
- Space calcium supplements for optimal absorption. Your body can best retain calcium in amounts of 500 mg or less. Figure out how many tablets (of 500 mg or less) you need to take through the day to get the recommended daily amount.
- Correct chronically low amounts of vitamin D and possibly magnesium; boron; fluoride; vitamins K, B12, and B6; and folic acid.
- Limit soft drinks because they are very high in phosphorus, which interferes with the ability to use calcium.
- Get the proper amount of vitamin D; the RDA is 400 IU. People who are housebound or live in northern climates with long winters can be at risk of vitamin D deficiency. Because vitamin D is potentially toxic, consuming intakes above the RDA is not recommended.
- Make regular weight-bearing exercise a part of your daily routine. Activities such as walking, jogging, bicycling, and skiing all stress the long bones of the body against the pull of gravity, thus strengthening your bones.
- Stop smoking. Smoking can be toxic to your bone cells. It can also reduce your body's absorption of calcium. Smokers also tend to maintain a lean body weight, experience menopause earlier, and show an accelerated rate of postmenopausal bone loss.
- Limit alcohol intake. Alcohol is thought to depress bone formation by directly reducing osteoblastic activity. Heavy drinkers usually do not have good eating habits and lack essential nutrients. Alcohol intoxication increases the risk of accidents and falls.

LINK UP to http://nof.org for the National Osteoporosis Foundation. They provide a huge variety of resources.

- Consider hormone replacement therapy if you are past menopause. Estrogen therapy reduces bone reabsorption and retards or halts postmenopausal bone loss. Even when started as late as six years after menopause, estrogen prevents further loss of bone mass but does not restore it to premenopausal levels.
- Moderate your caffeine intake. Caffeine can increase urinary calcium excretion. Heavy intake of beverages and foods containing caffeine along with poor calcium intake could compromise bone maintenance.
- Consider using certain herbal plants like kelp and other sea vegetables, as well as dandelion root, horsetail, and oat straw; these are good sources of calcium, magnesium, and trace minerals needed for strong and healthy bones. Kelp and other sea vegetables can be used as condiments to flavor food such as soups, casseroles, and salads.
- Try a chewable lactase supplement (such as Lactaid and Dairy Ease) just before you eat dairy foods if you're lactose intolerant.

INK UP to http://www.mayohealth.org to search for the latest studies, news releases, and links about osteoporosis from the Mayo Clinic's Health Oasis site.

Premenstrual Syndrome (PMS)

PMS is not a disease in the classic sense. More than 200 different symptoms have been reported by women in the days or weeks before their monthly menstrual periods. The most common symptoms include breast tenderness, abdominal bloating, weight gain, headaches, irritability, and food cravings.

Nutrition Issues

One factor that most women who suffer from PMS have in common is that they don't make smart food choices. PMS seems be one of those situations where marginal nutrient deficiencies add up to significant problems. Women who eat generous amount of nutrients from foods rarely suffer from symptoms of PMS or have milder symptoms if they do.

Dietary supplements and herbs have been a popular area for intervention. PMS is a miserable experience, and it's understandable that women will try most anything to get relief.

Selected Studies

Healthy, premenopausal women between the ages of 18 and 45 years who had moderate to severe, cyclically recurring premenstrual symptoms were recruited across the United States. The women were randomly assigned to receive 1,200 mg of elemental calcium per day in the form of calcium carbonate or placebo for three menstrual cycles. Of the 466 women who participated in the study, those who took the calcium supplements each day experienced a 48 percent reduction in their overall PMS symptoms, compared with a 30 percent reduction among women given dummy pills (*American Journal of Obstetrics and Gynecology,* August 1998). Calcium depletion may interact with female hormones at certain stages of the menstrual cycle, leading to the physical and emotional discomfort of PMS. But note that there was also a 30 percent reduction in symptoms in women who took the placebo.

New Nutrition *Recommendations for PMS*

- Get the nutrients you need from foods to compensate for the marginal deficiencies that make many women more prone to PMS.
- Break a sweat. Even moderate exercise can help reduce PMS symptoms. If you work up a sweat, the loss of water can help decrease bloating.
- Opt for high-carbohydrate foods like potatoes, whole-grain breads, or crackers instead of sweets. They'll help soothe your mood without aggravating your PMS symptoms.
- Watch your consumption of vitamin B_6; it is sometimes prescribed in toxic doses by gynecologists and other health care providers for relief of premenstrual syndrome symptoms. Don't exceed more than 50 mg/day or you are at risk for nerve damage.
- Limit consumption of alcohol, caffeine, and salt if these compounds aggravate your symptoms. Alcohol may worsen mood swings and irritability. Caffeine can increase breast tenderness and nervousness. Foods high in sodium may increase bloating and fluid retention.

Ulcers

Calming down and taking it easy isn't good advice for the prevention of ulcers. It's a myth that anxiety, anger, and type A personalities cause ulcers. Recent research shows that most ulcers are caused by the bacteria *Helicobacter pylori.* There are two main types of ulcers: duodenal and gastric. Duodenal ulcers are the more common variety and are located in the small intestine right next to the stomach. Gastric ulcers are true stomach ulcers that occur when stomach acid eats away at the stomach's lining. Esophageal ulcers are quite rare and are often a result of alcohol abuse.

It's believed that the *Helicobacter pylori* bacteria somehow change the tissue lining the digestive tract, making it more susceptible to ulcer formation. *Helicobacter pylori* is present in 92 percent of duodenal ulcers and 73 percent of gastric ulcers. Certain drugs can also promote the growth of ulcers. Aspirin and ibuprofen can irritate the stomach or intestinal lining enough to trigger an ulcer.

Fortunately, ulcers are relatively easy to treat; in many cases they are cured with antibiotics. Still, the dangers associated with ulcers—such as anemia, hemorrhage, pancreatic problems, and stomach cancer—are serious, so ulcers should always be monitored carefully.

Nutrition Issues
Overzealous use of over-the-counter analgesics (such as aspirin, ibuprofen, and naproxen), heavy alcohol use, and smoking exacerbate and may promote the development of ulcers. In fact, research indicates that heavy smokers are more prone to developing duodenal ulcers than are nonsmokers. Those who drink alcohol are more susceptible to esophageal ulcers. If you use moderate or great amounts of aspirin for a long period of time, you are at increased risk for gastric ulcers.

Studies show that gastric ulcers are more likely to develop in elderly people. This may be because arthritis is prevalent in the elderly, and alleviating arthritis pain often includes taking daily doses of aspirin or ibuprofen. Another contributing factor may be that with advancing age, the pylorus (the valve between the stomach and duodenum) relaxes and allows excess bile to seep into the stomach and erode the stomach lining.

Vitamins A and E and the mineral zinc help increase the production of mucin, a substance your body secretes to protect the stomach lining. Choosing more high-fiber foods can also reduce your chances of developing a duodenal ulcer. Fiber also enhances mucin secretion, which protects the duodenal lining.

For no known reason, people with type A blood are more likely to develop cancerous gastric ulcers. Duodenal ulcers tend to appear in people with type O blood.

New Nutrition *Recommendations for Ulcers*
- Ban bland diets. Since it's fairly clear that bacteria, not what you eat, cause most ulcers, there is no need to have a bland diet. There is no scientific evidence that a bland diet helps ulcers heal or reduces the painful symptoms that accompany ulcers.
- Don't overdose on iron supplements. Although people with bleeding ulcers can develop anemia and may need to take iron as a treatment, taking too much can irritate the stomach lining and make you worse. Ask your doctor how much iron you need.
- Avoid foods that irritate your stomach. Use common sense: if it upsets your stomach when you eat it, don't. Everyone is different, but spicy foods (especially black pepper and chili powder) and fatty foods are common irritants.
- Stop smoking. Heavy smokers are more likely to develop duodenal ulcers than nonsmokers, largely because nicotine is thought to prevent the pancreas from secreting acid-neutralizing enzymes.

- Don't eat close to bedtime. Late-night eating stimulates the secretion of stomach acid while you sleep.
- Cut out alcohol. It irritates the lining of the digestive tract. If you must drink, dilute with water, soda, or juice and eat food along with alcohol to help decrease its acid-stimulating effect.

10

Evaluating Nutrition Products and Purveyors

Accurate nutrition information is hard to obtain when your primary "scientific" source is your local newspaper, favorite magazine, Internet, or popular TV news/magazine show.

FREEDOM TO DECEIVE

> *"Congress shall make no law abridging the freedom of speech, or of the press."*
> —First Amendment to the U.S. Constitution

Freedom of expression is the right of every U.S. citizen. Each individual can gather and present or publish information or opinions without fear of punishment or control by the government. These freedoms apply to all types of printed and broadcast material, including seminars, books, newspapers, magazines, pamphlets, films, radio, and television programs. Why a review on constitutional freedoms? We all have the right to say or print anything. The only exceptions are very narrowly defined. If you don't threaten to overthrow the government, slander someone, or include pornographic material, you can publish your opinions on any topic as if they were fact. Legally, it doesn't matter if what you say is true or false. You can make things up, list impressive-sounding references that don't exist, and twist someone else's ideas or research. Just browse the diet and nutrition section of your local bookstore. Most of the offerings there should be shelved in the fiction section. Do any of these claims sound familiar?

- Lose as much weight as you want without depriving yourself
- Burn fat while you sleep
- Miracle diet pill lets you lose weight instantly

Most nutrition articles are written by journalists who write about science—not by scientists. Nutrition research today includes techniques and tools unknown a decade ago. Journalists may be excellent writers, but often they don't have the scientific savvy to critically examine the research behind the stories they write. Of course there are exceptions. If you rely on newspapers, here are some of the best journalists who currently cover nutrition topics: Nanci Helmich of *USA Today,* Jane Brody of the *New York Times,* Sally Squires of the *Washington Post,* Bob Condor of the *Chicago Tribune,* and Kathy Doheny who writes for the *L.A. Times.*

SIZING UP RESEARCH

People often ask why we need controlled clinical studies when it's so "obvious" that something has worked for years or centuries. The best answer is to look at studies that backfired. The 1992 CAST (Cardiac Arrhythmia Suppression Trial) study showed that commonly held beliefs are not always true. Three drugs were being routinely used in the 1980s and early 1990s to prevent irregular heartbeats (arrhythmia) in people after they had already had a heart attack. Researchers set up a study to determine which of the drugs was most effective. Fortunately, they included a control group in addition to the three "experimental" groups that received the various drugs. The control group didn't receive any medications to prevent arrhythmias, just a placebo (an inactive substance that looks the same as the medicine being tested). Guess what? Each of the three drugs being studied caused more deaths than the placebo. For years, physicians had routinely prescribed drugs they felt helped patients. Based on their experience, most physicians believed the drugs were helpful. If a carefully controlled study had not been done, no one would have ever realized these drugs were harming, not helping, people.

The Power of Placebo

If you feel better after using a product or having a procedure done, it is natural to credit the new pill, potion, or treatment. It is important to remember, however, that taking action often produces temporary relief of symptoms due to a placebo effect. This effect is a beneficial change that can't be explained by the treatment given. You don't even have to believe in the power of a placebo for it to work. The placebo effect may be enhanced by impressive procedures and an enthusiastic therapist or healer.

The placebo effect is inherently misleading. It can make you think something is effective when it's not. Without controlled clinical trials, any treatment that is used could receive credit for your body's natural ability to heal. Since placebo therapy does work sometimes, it's obvious that we need to learn more about how the mind and the spirit act to heal our bodies.

Sensationalized Science

In 1975 the chances were slim that a nutrition-related study published in a scientific journal would make the evening news or appear in the headlines of your morning newspaper. Just twenty-five years later, almost every

Wednesday or Thursday (the days most major medical journals release their articles to the media) it seems medical history is being made or rewritten.

There are many ways a scientific study can be completed, but none of them is perfect. Here are some of the most popular types.

Case-control studies try to match up people with similar profiles, except one of them has the active disease or ailment being studied and the other does not. The studies follow these sets of people over time to look for similarities and differences.

Clinical trials are usually short-term studies that provide different interventions to similar groups of people and compare differences or reactions.

Cohort studies start with basically healthy people and follow them over time, keeping track of their lifestyle patterns and rates of disease.

Epidemiological studies look at population trends and demographics to develop theories for noted changes or differences between people.

Prospective studies plan ahead for the variables they want to track over time and develop ways to collect that information.

Retrospective studies look at already accumulated study information and try to pull out information to reach conclusions that were not part of the original study design.

In May of 1996, two studies about sodium were published in the same week. One study in the *British Medical Journal* urged cutting back on salt, but research in the *Journal of the American Medical Association* (*JAMA*) proclaimed no need for concern about salt intake. Then in March of 1998, research papers on both sides of the ocean flip-flopped positions. Another British journal, *Lancet,* reported that people with low sodium intakes had higher death rates and questioned the recommendation to reduce salt intake for the whole population. On the U.S. side, a major controlled trial of sodium restriction in older people with high blood pressure, in the March 1998 issue of *JAMA,* provided clear evidence of the benefit of decreased salt intake in this group. The *JAMA* article said that a decrease in salt intake, especially if combined with weight reduction, had definite benefits, such as preventing cardiovascular complications or reducing the need for drug treatment for hypertensive men and women ages 60 to 80.

Confused yet? First of all, each of these studies deals with different issues. The 1998 studies were looking at different groups of people in markedly different ways. The British researchers were questioning the need to restrict salt intake for the population at large. They did suggest that one shortcoming in their research can't be overlooked: some of the people in their study who died may have been on a low-sodium diet because of existing cardiovascular disease. Their study didn't exclude such people, who have higher death rates. The second 1998 study focused on a specific subgroup—older people with high blood pressure. If you are between 60 and 80 years old and have high blood pressure, a low-sodium diet is usually a good thing. Unfortunately, because of the misleading and conflicting headlines, a person with heart disease, severe high blood pressure, or certain forms of liver or kidney disease may consider dropping low-salt diet. That action could be dangerous or even deadly. Never change how you eat based on just one or two studies, especially if you've only heard of them through the media.

As you wait in the check-out lane at the supermarket, tabloid papers and popular women's magazines shout dramatic claims and amazing health findings that often contradict each other. You need to look beyond the hyped-up headlines and catchy phrases for the truth.

Rating Magazines for Accuracy

The American Council on Science and Health (ACSH) has been tracking magazine nutrition reporting for fifteen years. Here are their most recent findings.

Magazine	Percent Accurate Nutrition Information	Magazine	Percent Accurate Nutrition Information
Consumer Reports	95	Redbook	83
Better Homes and Gardens	92	Runner's World	82
Good Housekeeping	90	Shape	81
Glamour	89	Men's Health	81
Parents	88	Fitness	79
Health	87	Mademoiselle	79
Reader's Digest	86	Self	77
Prevention	86	Cosmopolitan	74
Woman's Day	85	Muscle & Fitness	70
Cooking Light	85	New Woman	69
McCall's	83		

Source: ACSH Nutrition Accuracy in *Popular Magazines Special Report,* 1995–1996

Don't Swallow Half-Baked Nutrition Claims

First of all, never change your lifestyle habits based on a single study or report. If you've ever worked in communications, you'll realize how easy it is to get the facts wrong. Remember the "Liquid Candy" report from the

Center for Science in the Public Interest (CSPI) in the fall of 1998? It announced a dramatic increase in teen consumption of soft drinks. Two weeks after the report was highlighted by nationwide media, it was discovered that a consulting firm hired by CSPI made a serious error in calculation. It failed to divide the number of cans of pop consumed over two days by two to get a daily average intake. The corrected press release listed thirty-six separate mistakes from ten different sections of the original report, including additional mistakes made by CSPI. If you never saw the corrections from this report, you are not alone.

You don't have to be a health statistician (though it would help) to objectively dissect a scientific study. There are lots of simple ways to determine if the conclusions of research are valid and if they apply to you. Using five key factors, let's size up the much-publicized *Journal of the American Medical Association* study from the Arizona Cancer Institute that suggests selenium supplements can reduce the risk of many different types of cancer.

1. Study size: 1,300

2. Study group: men (75 percent) and women (25 percent); all people with a previous history of skin cancer who live in the southeastern United States

3. Length of the study: 4 years

4. Study objective: To determine if selenium supplements can help protect against skin cancer

5. Control group protocol: Half the group took 200 mcg of selenium and the other half took placebos. Neither the subjects nor the researchers knew who had the placebo.

Size: The number of subjects in this study is too small to prove there is a cancer-reduction benefit from selenium supplements. Many impressive statistics are quoted, such as: the selenium group developed 63 percent fewer prostate cancers, 58 percent fewer colorectal cancers, and 46 percent fewer lung cancers than the placebo group. How many new cancers would you normally expect 1,300 people to be diagnosed with over four years time? If a specific cancer commonly affects 1 in 1,000 people, then you need large numbers of people in both control and experimental groups to know if your results are significant. How many people who have already been treated for skin cancer go on to develop a completely different type of the disease? That factor increases the pool of needed test subjects even more.

Study group: Just 25 percent of the participants were women (about 325 females), not nearly enough to estimate how selenium supplements affect women in general. Also, women cannot get prostate cancer and have much lower rates of colorectal cancer than men. Don't forget that all the participants had a history of skin cancer—do you? These people live in the southwestern part of the United States, where foods are often low in selenium. That's because the soil in this part of the country is low in selenium. Do you live in the scorching Southwest? If not, you're different from the study group and the results may not apply to you. Environmental conditions like sun exposure surely contributed to the risk of their initial skin cancer.

Length of the study: In an ideal world, long-term studies that span the course of generations would be used to draw scientific conclusions. Realistically, we don't want to wait that long for cures to dangerous and debilitating conditions. There needs to be a middle ground. How reasonable is it to expect that in any four-year period, someone would develop cancer? Would longer-term supplementation show the same or different effects? Most research concludes by asking more questions than it answers.

Study objective: The original clinical trial was to determine if selenium affected risk of skin cancer. The answer to the original study question— Do selenium supplements protect against skin cancer?—was no. It wasn't until the study had been under way for several years that the scientists decided to start looking at whether selenium supplements had an impact on cancers other than skin cancer. Such unplanned searches are mathematically more likely to turn up results that occur by chance.

Control group: Controlling people isn't easy. It's important that no one involved directly in the study knows who gets the "real" medicine and who doesn't. Care must be taken to be sure that both placebo and the pills, potions, or remedies look, smell, taste, or feel identical. For example, zinc lozenges taste terrible. Placebo zinc lozenges should taste just as bad. That's because study participants often talk with each other and the study staff. They like to compare notes while waiting for appointments.

How is compliance tracked? Did the people in the study really take all the pills they were supposed to? Did they also take other products and not inform the researchers? Often, people who participate in clinical trials are paid. In addition, they may receive free medical care, in-depth laboratory tests, gain important information about their health, and receive much personal attention. Sometimes these benefits are enough to "fake" compliance. Food-related studies are even more difficult to control. How accurately and honestly do you think people estimate and record the types and amount of food they eat?

Funding sources: Everyone loves to zero in on who funded the study. It's a reasonable concern. Think of it like buying a car from a used-car salesperson. You need to approach with caution and ask lots of questions. Most research is funded by private companies. If we relied solely on federal dollars, little valuable research would occur. For many pharmaceutical companies, research is part of their business. Now that foods are being investigated for their health benefits, it makes sense that food companies and dietary supplement manufacturers will start funding research, too.

Also, beware of consumer groups that publicize opinions as fact. Just because an agency is nonprofit doesn't mean it is ethical. Nonprofit companies need money to operate just like for-profit companies. Nonprofit companies just have different tax advantages and must spend most of the money they take in instead of rewarding owners or shareholders.

Junk Science

Any combination of the following signs should raise a red flag of warning to be skeptical.

1. recommendations that promise a quick fix

2. dire warnings of danger from a single product or regimen

3. claims that sound too good to be true

4. simplistic conclusions drawn from a complex study

5. recommendations based on a single study

6. dramatic statements that are refuted by reputable scientific organizations

7. lists of "good" and "bad" foods

8. recommendations made to help sell a product

9. recommendations based on studies published without peer review

10. recommendations from studies that ignore differences among individuals or groups

Source: Food and Nutrition Science Alliance (FANSA), a partnership of The American Dietetic Association, American Society for Clinical Nutrition, American Society for Nutritional Sciences, and Institute of Food Technologists

SUPPLEMENT SAVVY

Have you ever ventured into a casino? Dim lights, smoky air, and a rainbow of flashy games entice you to part with your money. You might wonder if the slots are rigged or the dealers crooked; yet the seductive promise of walking away a winner can be difficult to resist. This same image comes to mind when stalking the supplement shelves. Though the lighting is better and smoking is prohibited, you usually don't know what you're getting into, but hopes are high for choosing a winner.

Although most people believe otherwise, vitamin, mineral, herbal, and other dietary supplements are some of the most loosely regulated products in America. In 1994, over 2 million Americans wrote or called congressional representatives and told them to back off on supplement regulations being proposed by the Dietary Supplement Health and Education Act (DSHEA). Supplement manufacturers misled people into thinking that all dietary supplements would become as regulated as prescription drugs—in other words, limited or difficult to get. The public confusion and upset led to passage of a flimsy set of regulations that fail to provide even minimum standards of safety and truthfulness. Instead of requiring that all types of supplements be proven safe and effective, as is required for foods, drugs, and additives, the Food and Drug Administration (FDA) must wait for proof that a product has caused serious harm or death before it can be pulled from the shelves.

DSHEA essentially gives dietary supplement manufacturers freedom to market more products as dietary supplements and provide information about their products' benefits on the label. No license, inspection, or quality control is mandated. There are no government specifications for scientific testing of supplements. Each manufacturer can determine what type of testing, if any, will be done. Dosages are also set by product manufacturers, not the FDA.

Supplement manufacturers aren't required to completely list the ingredients included in their products. For example, researchers at Cedars-Sinai Bone Center in Los Angeles found that 10 percent of the older people they studied were taking toxic levels of vitamin D. Two of the supplements commonly used by those in the study (which happened to contain some of the highest levels of vitamin D) didn't even list vitamin D as an ingredient! Another example is of a weight lifter disqualified from international competition because he had ephedrine (a potentially harmful stimulant) in his system. In protest over the results of his drug screening test, he sent his regular supplements to a laboratory for analysis. It was discovered that indeed the manufacturer had included ephedrine (a banned substance) in a supplement without listing it on the ingredient label.

The United States Pharmacopoeia (USP) sets standards for drug products. They recently established standards for individual and combination vitamin and mineral nutritional supplements. These standards detail quality practices for supplement manufacturers. Because the USP is a nongovernmental organization, compliance with such standards is voluntary for supplements. However, USP standards for drug products are legally enforceable by the FDA. The USP notation on supplement labels is currently the best way ensure product quality.

There are several key measures that are important in making sure that vitamin and mineral tablets and capsules do the job you expect them to. The following quality indicators are based on USP laboratory testing standards:

- **Disintegration** measures how fast a tablet or capsule breaks into small pieces. Smaller piece size makes it easier for the ingredients to dissolve. If a tablet or capsule does not break down within a certain amount of time, it may pass through your body without being absorbed. Water-soluble vitamins should disintegrate in less than forty-five minutes (uncoated) or in less than sixty minutes (coated).
- **Dissolution** gauges how fast and how much of a vitamin or mineral dissolves in a fluid that is similar to your digestive tract. USP standards track pyridoxine when testing multivitamins. Their standards require that 75 percent be dissolved within sixty minutes.
- **Strength** is the amount of a specific vitamin or mineral substance in each tablet or capsule. To meet USP product quality standards, the amount present must be within a narrow range of the amount declared on the label.
- **Purity** is controlled by USP standards that set a range for acceptable impurities that can result from contamination or degradation of the product during processing or storage.
- **Expiration dates** must be imprinted on the package. When the date is past due, the nutrient ingredients in a bottle or package of supplements may no longer meet USP standards of purity, strength, and/or quality.

It's been widely reported that you can test your own supplements at home for disintegration. But home experiments using water or vinegar don't come close to copying the conditions in your stomach or at a laboratory.

The Claim Game

DSHEA allows all types of vitamin, mineral, herbal, and dietary supplements to carry "structure or function" claims, but not statements that imply their products can treat, diagnose, cure, or prevent disease. All structure or function claims must be based on scientific information about using supplements to maintain health. However, the term "scientific" is defined by the supplement manufacturer or the advertising agency. Thumb through magazine ads for supplements and you'll see that almost anything counts as scientific in the minds of the companies that are challenged to market these products.

Benefit claims have always been a controversial feature of dietary supplement labeling, and manufacturers rely on claims to sell products. Can you trust them? DSHEA and previous food labeling laws allow supplement manufacturers to use three types of claims. Nutrient content claims and health claims follow rules similar to those required for food products. Nutrition support claims, which include "structure-function claims," are unique to supplement products. As with food products, nutrient levels required for any claims are based on Daily Values and not Recommended Dietary Allowances.

Nutrient-content claims describe the level of a nutrient in a food or dietary supplement. For example, a supplement containing at least 200 mg of calcium per serving could carry the claim "high in calcium" since it provides at least 20 percent of the DV for calcium. A supplement with at least 12 mg per serving of vitamin C could state on its label "Excellent source of vitamin C."

Health claims indicate a link between a food or substance and a disease or health-related condition. The FDA preauthorizes these claims based on a review of the scientific evidence or authoritative statements from certain scientific bodies, such as the National Academy of Sciences, that show or describe a well-established diet-to-health link. As of this writing, a few of the approved claims that appropriate supplements may use include:

- folic acid and a decreased risk of neural tube defect–affected pregnancy (if the supplement contains sufficient amounts of folic acid)
- calcium and a lower risk of osteoporosis (if the supplement contains sufficient amounts of calcium)
- psyllium seed disease (if the supplement contains sufficient amounts of psyllium seed husk) husk and a lower risk of coronary heart (as part of a diet low in cholesterol and saturated fat)

Examples of prohibited claims for a dietary supplement include "protects against cancer," "treats hot flashes," and "reduces nausea associated with chemotherapy." If you find dietary supplements whose labels state or imply that the product can help diagnose, treat, cure, or prevent a disease (e.g., "cures cancer" or "treats arthritis"), remember that the product is being marketed illegally as a drug and has not been evaluated for safety or effectiveness.

Nutrition support claims describe a link between a nutrient and the deficiency disease that can result if the nutrient is lacking in the diet. For example, an iron supplement label could state that iron prevents anemia. When these types of claims are used, the label must mention the prevalence of the nutrient-deficiency disease in the United States. Structure-function claims refer to the supplement's effect on the body's structure or function, including its overall effect on a person's well-being. Examples of structure-function claims are:

- calcium builds strong bones
- antioxidants maintain cell integrity
- fiber maintains bowel regularity

Manufacturers can use structure-function claims without FDA authorization. Structure-function claims are easy to spot because the label must carry the disclaimer "This statement has not been evaluated by the Food and Drug Administration. This product is not intended to diagnose, treat, cure, or prevent any disease."

In an effort to correct problems with supplement regulations, the FDA is trying to update DSHEA. "Consumers want access to dietary supplements, but also need reliable information about the products they are consuming," announced William Schultz, the FDA's Deputy Commissioner for Policy, in explaining the proposed changes. "By clarifying for manufacturers what types of claims can and cannot be made on a dietary supplement label, this new proposal helps consumers make more informed and wiser choices."

ANATOMY OF THE NEW REQUIREMENTS FOR DIETARY SUPPLEMENT LABELS

Information that was first required on supplement labels in March 1999 includes:

- statement of identity (e.g., "vitamin C")

- net quantity of contents (e.g., "100 capsules")

- optional structure-function claim must include the warning "This statement has not been evaluated by the Food and Drug Administration. This product is not intended to diagnose, treat, cure, or prevent any disease."

- directions for use (e.g., "Take one capsule daily")

- supplement facts panel (lists serving size, amount, and active ingredient)

- other ingredients in descending order of predominance and by common name or proprietary blend

- name and place of business of manufacturer, packer, or distributor. This is the address to write for more product information.

Source: Adapted from *FDA Consumer,* September/October 1998

HOW TO READ A SUPPLEMENT LABEL

This is the brand name of the product

"Serving size" is the manufacturer's suggested serving expressed in the appropriate unit (tablet, capsule, softgel, packet, teaspoonful)

"Amount Per Tablet" heads the listing of nutrients contained in the supplement, followed by the quantity present in each tablet or capsule (if the serving size is one tablet).

International Unit (I.U.) is a standard unit of measurement for fat-soluble vitamins (A, D, and E)

Milligram (mg) and microgram (mcg) are units of measurement for water-soluble vitamins (C and B-complex) and minerals. A milligram is equal to 1/1000 of a gram (a microgram is equal to 1/1,000 of a milligram).

A complete list of all ingredients will appear outside the Nutrition Facts box. This includes nutrients and other ingredients used to formulate the supplement, in decreasing order by weight.

This voluntary notation indicates the supplement has passed certain quality control tests.

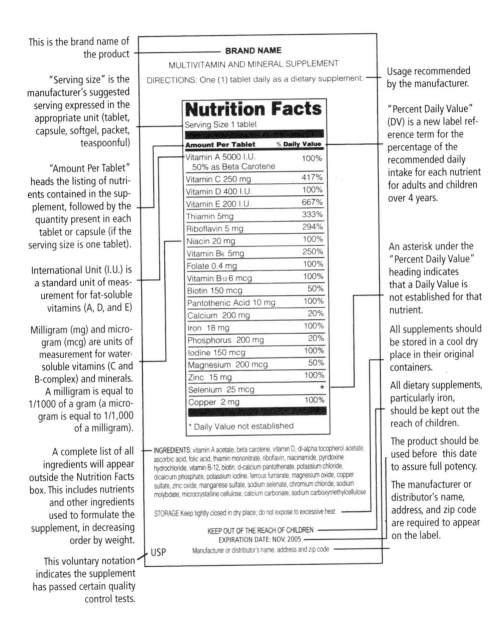

BRAND NAME

MULTIVITAMIN AND MINERAL SUPPLEMENT

DIRECTIONS: One (1) tablet daily as a dietary supplement.

Nutrition Facts
Serving Size 1 tablet

Amount Per Tablet	% Daily Value
Vitamin A 5000 I.U. 50% as Beta Carotene	100%
Vitamin C 250 mg	417%
Vitamin D 400 I.U.	100%
Vitamin E 200 I.U.	667%
Thiamin 5mg	333%
Riboflavin 5 mg	294%
Niacin 20 mg	100%
Vitamin B6 5mg	250%
Folate 0.4 mg	100%
Vitamin B12 6 mcg	100%
Biotin 150 mcg	50%
Pantothenic Acid 10 mg	100%
Calcium 200 mg	20%
Iron 18 mg	100%
Phosphorus 200 mg	20%
Iodine 150 mcg	100%
Magnesium 200 mcg	50%
Zinc 15 mg	100%
Selenium 25 mcg	*
Copper 2 mg	100%

* Daily Value not established

INGREDIENTS: vitamin A acetate, beta carotene, vitamin D, dl-alpha tocopherol acetate, ascorbic acid, folic acid, thiamin mononitrate, riboflavin, niacinamide, pyridoxine hydrochloride, vitamin B-12, biotin. d-calcium pantothenate, potassium chloride, dicalcium phosphate, potassium iodine. ferrous fumarate, magnesium oxide, copper sulfate, zinc oxide, manganese sulfate, sodium selenate, chromium chloride, sodium molybdate, microcrystalline cellulose, calcium carbonate, sodium carboxymethylcellulose

STORAGE Keep tightly closed in dry place; do not expose to excessive heat.

KEEP OUT OF THE REACH OF CHILDREN
EXPIRATION DATE: NOV. 2005
Manufacturer or distributor's name, address and zip code

USP

Usage recommended by the manufacturer.

"Percent Daily Value" (DV) is a new label reference term for the percentage of the recommended daily intake for each nutrient for adults and children over 4 years.

An asterisk under the "Percent Daily Value" heading indicates that a Daily Value is not established for that nutrient.

All supplements should be stored in a cool dry place in their original containers.

All dietary supplements, particularly iron, should be kept out the reach of children.

The product should be used before this date to assure full potency.

The manufacturer or distributor's name, address, and zip code are required to appear on the label.

The Federal Trade Commission (FTC), not the FDA, regulates claims made in the advertising of dietary supplements. In recent years, the FTC has taken a number of enforcement actions against companies whose advertisements contained false and misleading information. Erroneous claims that chromium picolinate was a treatment for weight loss and high blood cholesterol were removed. An action in 1997 targeted ads for an ephedrine alkaloid supplement because they understated the degree of the product's risk and featured a man falsely described as a doctor.

According to many professional groups, including the American Dietetic Association, consumer perception of supplement claims should also be part of the decision-making process. For instance, just what does "strengthen immunity" mean to the average supplement shopper? Preliminary research by the FDA shows that current health claims lead consumers to believe that products are likely to have positive health effects well beyond those promoted on the label.

In 1999, the Federal Trade Commission released a business guide for the dietary supplement industry. It encourages the industry to use accurate information in making claims. For the first time ever, it's spelled out that anyone who "participates directly or indirectly in the marketing of dietary supplements has an obligation to make sure that claims are presented truthfully and to check the adequacy of the support." According to the FTC, the amount and type of support needed will depend on a variety of factors. These factors include consumers' expectation of what a claim means, the specific claim being made, how claims are presented in the context of the entire ad, and how statements are qualified. In evaluating the adequacy of support for a claim, the FTC expects to consult with experts in a wide variety of fields, including those with a background in botanicals and traditional medicine. The FTC's definition of dietary supplements includes vitamins, minerals, herbal products, hormones, and amino acids.

SUPPLEMENT PROFITEERS

It's not just the claims that are sometimes fraudulent, often it's also the prices. In May 1999, the U.S. Justice Department won its largest case ever, with fines of $725 million, against several giant foreign drug and chemical companies for engaging in a worldwide conspiracy to raise and fix the prices of vitamins and other supplements. It's estimated that the inflated prices in effect since January of 1990 affected more than $5 billion of common products ranging from vitamins to enriched foods, including milk, cereal, and pet foods. The firms involved include Hoffman-LaRoche, BASF AG, and Lonza AG. More charges are expected to be filed as the case progresses.

The U.S. market for vitamins and supplements is projected to be worth between $11 billion and $20 billion. The editor of *Nutrition Business Journal* estimates that mainstream physicians directly sold about $120 million worth of supplements to their patients last year. Chiropractors, homeopaths, naturopaths, and other alternative practitioners sold $680 million in supplements from their offices.

For years the federal government has frowned upon doctors sending patients' blood and urine samples to their own labs for analysis. The concern is that extra tests will be ordered to add profits to the balance sheet. The American Medical Association Code of Medical Ethics says physicians should not let their wallets influence what they prescribe. Would you trust a doctor who recommended supplements if he or she made as much or more money from selling supplements as from an office visit?

Personal selling creates the lion's share of wealth in the supplement industry. Pyramid selling programs like Amway, Rexall, and Shaklee allow anyone to sell supplements. These salespeople benefit personally when you take their advice, as does the eager health food store employee who works on commission. If you've ever been asked to sell supplements, you are probably aware that more time and energy goes into training you to be a super salesperson than teaching you about what you sell.

If you are spending more than $10 a month on vitamin/mineral supplements, you're getting ripped off. Enough said.

PROTECTING YOUR INVESTMENT

Ads for supplements have powerful messages that play on your fears and exploit the desire to find an easy and "natural" solution to eating right. The FDA has little control over dietary supplements. This means that you have the responsibility for checking on the safety of dietary supplements and determining the truthfulness of any label claims.

Here's how to get the most for your money when purchasing vitamin/mineral supplements:

- Choose only vitamin/mineral supplements designated as meeting USP guidelines to ensure you are getting a quality product that will deliver what's listed on the label.
- Don't pay extra for "natural" supplements—they all work the same. Minerals are always natural since they can't be made from other substances. Vitamins present in food and plants are considered natural vitamins. Vitamins created in a laboratory are synthetic. There is no difference in most vitamin molecules whether they are synthetic or natural. Synthetic vitamins are usually less expensive, their potency can be better controlled, and they may be purer or less

contaminated with pesticides and fertilizers. On the other hand, natural vitamins may, by default, include other food components that are beneficial to health. One notable exception to this rule is vitamin E. The natural form of vitamin E (alpha-tocopherol) varies slightly from the synthetic versions (beta-, delta-, and gamma-tocopherol) and the nutrient is more effective in the natural form.

- Compare the labels. Generics can be a good deal. National retailers like K-Mart, Target, and Wal-Mart purchase supplements that are often identical to the higher-priced name brands.

- Don't pay extra for high-potency supplements. Since "high potency" is not legally defined, anyone can slap the term of the label of a supplement. It means nothing. Supplements work best when taken in several small doses spread throughout the day. That's because you can absorb more of a nutrient when your system isn't overloaded. When a high concentration of a nutrient enters your bloodstream, your kidneys work to quickly get rid of the excess. Taking a one-shot supplement isn't ideal, but it is convenient. Time-release supplements don't offer much of an advantage. Since vitamins and minerals are absorbed at different places in the gastrointestinal tract, it's highly unlikely that a time-release tablet will deliver each nutrient at the optimal time and place for absorption. Vitamin sprays and patches are sold in some parts of the United States and Canada. Contrary to their marketing literature, it has not been proven that you can absorb more nutrients because they have been applied to your skin or sprayed inside your mouth.

- Take your multiple vitamin and mineral supplements with food and water. You need fat and water to maximize nutrient absorption.

- Avoid frills and extras such as glandular products, hormones, and amino acids. All of these add-ons can increase the cost of a supplement without a proven benefit. Supplements that include such products often do not completely label or disclose the total amounts of nutrients they contain and may result in potentially toxic doses.

- Never purchase supplements past their expiration dates, no matter how cheap they are. In fact, if a product is within six months of expiring you can be sure it's lost some of its stability and potency.

- Never store supplements anywhere in your bathroom. The heat and moisture variations may change the action of the vitamin or speed deterioration. Store supplements tightly capped and safely out of the reach of young children. Most supplements do best in a cool, dry place away from direct sunlight. A high shelf in the kitchen—away from the oven or stove—is usually a good choice.

- If money is scarce, spend it on produce instead of supplements. Eating a variety of wholesome foods has a greater benefit than supplements to correct poor nutritional status.

ALTERNATIVE TO WHAT?

In 1993, a landmark study captured attention for today's alternative medicine movement. It was published in the prestigious *New England Journal of Medicine*. News stories based on this article proclaimed everyone was jumping into alternative medicine. It made you think What am I missing out on?

Dr. David Eisenberg wrote a special article (not a clinical research paper), "Unconventional Medicine in the United States, Prevalence, Costs and Patterns of Use." The paper compiled results of a random telephone survey of 1,539 consumers. The survey included only those out of 2,295 households contacted where someone actually answered all of the questions asked. People were excluded who did not speak English, were physically or mentally incapacitated, refused to participate, or hung up before finishing the survey. When the participants indicated they had a "bothersome or serious" health problem, they were asked if they had seen their doctor for this condition in the last twelve months. Next, they were asked if they had used "any other kinds of therapies and treatments." A list of sixteen unconventional therapies was read for each ailment that was noted. The person would say if they had tried each one. Here's the list in order of most frequently reported therapies:

- relaxation techniques
- chiropractic
- massage
- imagery
- spiritual healing
- commercial weight-loss program
- lifestyle diets
- herbal medicine
- megavitamin therapy
- self-help groups
- energy healing
- biofeedback
- hypnosis
- homeopathy
- acupuncture
- folk remedies

These sixteen categories included any common option for improving health, such as joining a Weight Watchers group, trying a low-fat diet, napping for relaxation, joining a support group, having a massage, trying to be positive about feeling better, or taking anything more than a one-a-day multivitamin supplement. Newspaper headlines screamed, "One in Three People Use Alternative Medicine." The fire was lit.

In fairness to Dr. Eisenberg and his colleagues, their conclusions were quite different from the media reports. The researchers summarized: "Our observation that the majority of users of unconventional therapy did not discuss this therapy with their medical doctors suggests a deficiency in current patient-doctor relations. Medical doctors should begin to ask their patients about their use of unconventional therapy whenever they obtain a history. We suggest that medical schools include information about unconventional therapies and the clinical social sciences (anthropology and sociology) in their curriculums." This conclusion isn't news. Sometimes health care providers are so focused on the disease they forget there is a human being to interact with. Have you ever heard a doctor or nurse talk about the "appendix in room 202" or the "broken arm in exam room 3"?

Perhaps physicians should begin to view diet, nutrition, relaxation, massage therapy, and referral to self-help and support groups as not only conventional but essential therapy for people with chronic health problems. There is increasing scientific support for the benefit of such changes in lifestyle.

EXPERT EVALUATION

If you have a chronic disease, complicated eating preferences, or just like the idea of checking out your food intake, it's critical to find a reputable professional to help guide you. As with all trades or professions there is a range of competencies among those who practice. Team up with someone who has a strong academic and practical background in food, nutrition, and health. They should be able to personalize suggestions and offer strategies right for you.

Memorizing the chemical structures of vitamins or digestive pathways doesn't make someone a nutrition expert. Many health professionals, including doctors and nurses, learn the biology of nutrition. Most don't have a clue how to translate that into what to eat in order to attain optimal health. The endorsement of special diets or nutrition products by people with a string of initials after their name should make you skeptical. Nutrition professionals shouldn't be endorsing specific products. Don't hand over your money to hucksters and celebrities, they may be great salespeople, but they are not usually great nutrition advisors.

Who's Who in Nutrition

Registered Dietitian (RD)

No doubt about it, RDs are the nutrition experts in the United States. No other group of individuals has their integrated training in the art and science of food and nutrition. An RD separates fact from fiction. He or she can explain the latest scientific findings in an easy-to-understand way. An RD gives you personal attention and helps you create an eating pattern and nutrition program that is uniquely yours.

RDs must complete a bachelor's or master's degree in nutrition, dietetics, public health, biochemistry, medicine, or other nutrition specialty from an accredited college or university. As part of, or in addition to, this schooling, RDs must perform a rigorous, supervised internship. When the learning and practice are completed, there's a national exam to pass. Continuing professional education is mandatory for RDs. The only credible national credential for a nutrition expert is the RD.

ANDY HOTLINE to the National Center for Nutrition and Dietetics is 1-800-366-1655. You can ask to be referred to a registered dietitian in your area.

INK UP to a registered dietitian at **http://www.eatright.org** at the American Dietetic Association.

Nutritionist

Never see a nutritionist. That's because anyone can claim this title. No credentials, no knowledge or training, no ethics required. The term "nutritionist" is not federally regulated and neither are its practitioners. If someone calls him- or herself a nutritionist, ask what other credentials he or she has. Some RDs may also refer to themselves as nutritionists. Be sure to verify the RD status.

Certified Nutritional Consultant (CNC)

The trademark designation CNC after a nutritional consultant's name indicates the person is a member of the American Association of Nutritional Consultants (AANC). Being a member or certified member of this association doesn't mean you're qualified to practice nutrition. "Membership in AANC and its predecessors has been open to anyone" according to Dr. Stephen Barrett, a leading authority on medical fraud. To prove that fact, years ago, Victor Herbert, M.D., J.D., a prominent nutrition scientist, obtained a "professional membership" for his dog in AANC by sending $50 plus the name and address of his pet. Today's fees are higher, $150, plus you are required to take an open-book, at-home exam. But according to AANC's web site, "we realize that after looking over the tests, the candidate may feel that he or she needs to review one or more of the subjects. Therefore, we include with the examination a list of recommended textbooks. The textbooks recommended are those which will assist the candidate in successfully completing the specific portions of the examination the candidate finds troubling." Enough said.

ALTERNATIVE SYSTEMS OF PRACTICE

The Office of Alternative Medicine (OAM) was initiated by congressional mandate under the 1992 National Institutes of Health (NIH) appropriations bill. The mission was to oversee new types of medical practices and provide grant money for their research. Questionable leadership and funding of inappropriate projects quickly eroded political and public confidence in this agency. In 1998 the OAM was reorganized as the National Center for Complementary and Alternative Medicine (NCCAM). The NCCAM's purpose is to facilitate the evaluation of alternative medicine treatment modalities and provide a public information clearinghouse. It does not serve as a referral agency for alternative medical treatment or individual practitioners.

The NCCAM has funded nine Specialty Research Centers to study complementary and alternative treatments for specific health conditions. These centers form the foundation for conducting ongoing research through the NIH. Current NCCAM Specialty Research Centers and their study specialties include:

HANDY HOTLINE to the NCCAM is 888-644-6226 for inquiries about NCCAM research and general information about complementary and alternative medicine.

Minneapolis Medical Research Foundation: Addictions

Columbia University: Aging and women's health

University of Maryland School of Medicine: Arthritis

University of Michigan Taubman Health Care Center: Cardiovascular disease

Maharishi University of Management: Cardiovascular disease and aging in African Americans

Palmer Center for Chiropractic Research: Chiropractic

Kaiser Foundation Hospitals: Craniofacial disorders

Oregon Health Sciences University: Neurological disorders

University of Arizona Health Sciences Center: Pediatrics

LINK UP to http://nccam.nih.gov/ for more detailed information on research studies in progress and background on the OAM and NCCAM.

Surfing the Net

The amount of nutrition information available via computer is mind boggling. With so much data, the challenge is finding trustworthy sites to meet your needs. All of the web links listed in each chapter have been accessed just prior to publication to help ensure they are current. They have not been screened for accuracy, just for the specific web address (URL) listed. If you want to check out other sites, you might start with the Tufts University Nutrition Navigator (http://www.navigator.tufts.edu). This site evaluates the accuracy of several web sites and allows you to do a keyword search or search across eight categories:

- educators
- general nutrition
- health professionals
- journalists
- kids
- parents
- special dietary needs
- women

The Nutrition Navigator's in-depth reviews are based on criteria developed by an advisory board of leading U.S. and Canadian nutrition experts and conducted by RDs at Tufts. Sites are rated on a 25-point scale. Each site can score up to 10 points for accuracy, 7 points for depth of nutrition information, 3 points for frequency of updates, and 5 points for ease of use. Sites with accuracy scores below 7 are not recommended. Why? "If a site isn't based on sound science, it doesn't matter how good it is in other ways. Our goal is to help people get to the information they can trust most," says Jeanne Goldberg, Ph.D., RD, director of the Center on Nutrition Communication at the Tufts University School of Nutrition Science and Policy.

The U.S. Food and Drug Administration (FDA) is one of the main government organizations that posts nutrition and health information for both consumers and health professionals. According to William M. Rados, director of communications staff at the Office of Public Affairs at the FDA, "We're actually doing away with print distribution of many materials and relying on the Internet instead." The Electronic Freedom of Information Act Amendments of 1996 requires all federal agencies to post any document on the Web that would normally be posted in reading rooms or requested by more than one person.

INK UP to **http://www.fda.gov** to access a variety of food and nutrition resources from the Food and Drug Administration.

With more than sixty central web sites on eight different domains, the Department of Health and Human Services (HHS) provides one of the richest and most reliable sources of health information on the Internet.

INK UP to http://www.nlm.nih.gov for Healthfinder, a gateway site to help consumers find health and human services information quickly. Healthfinder includes links to more than 1,250 web sites, including federal, state, local, non-profit, university, and other consumer health resources. Topics are organized by subject in an index.

INK UP to http://www.nlm.nih.gov for Medline, the world's most extensive collection of published medical information, coordinated by the National Library of Medicine. Originally designed for health professionals and researchers, Medline is also ideal for students and those seeking more specific or technical information about health conditions and treatment. Once a fee-based service, Medline is now free. PubMed provides direct web links between Medline abstracts and the publishers of the original full-text articles.

INK UP to http://www.nih.gov/health/ for the NIH Health Information Page, which provides access to the National Institutes of Health consumer health information resources including publications, clearinghouses, and databases.

HOW TO DUCK THE QUACKS

"Americans love hogwash—in the sense that 'hogwash' is worthless, false, or ridiculous speech or writing," said Edward H. Rynearson, M.D., Emeritus Professor of Medicine of the Mayo Clinic and Mayo Foundation, at the Scientific Awards Dinner at a meeting of the American Medical Association on June 26, 1973. Not much has changed since then. Nutrition quackery today mimics the patent medicine craze of the 1800s. Early patent medicines were imported from Europe and sold by postmasters, goldsmiths, grocers, and tailors. Many of the patent medicine manufacturers were the first companies to seek national audiences through daily newspapers and national weeklies to get their product messages out to the public. "Lydia Pinkham's Vegetable Compound" was the most successful patent medicine of the nineteenth century. She had special cures to heal a variety of "women's ills." Grain alcohol was the largest ingredient of most patent medicines, including Pinkham's. In addition to the vegetable extracts and sugar that gave each brand its flavor and color, the remedies were sometimes laced with cocaine, caffeine, opium, or morphine. The Sears catalog sold a morphine-laced mixture intended to be slipped into a wayward husband's coffee in order to keep him home nights. Bored house-wives and the homebound elderly were susceptible to becoming patent medicine addicts. Other patent medicines included "Kopp's Baby Friend," which was made of sweetened water and morphine, and was advertised as the perfect way to calm babies down. Or wives could try Dr. Winslow's Soothing Syrup on husbands who like to roam at night. It promised to "make 'em lay like the dead 'til mornin'."

Nutty Nutritionists

Adelle Davis sold more than 10 million copies of her four books, includ-ing *Let's Get Well.* Much of what she said remains true: our diets are loaded with too much salt, sugar, and preservatives. Despite a degree in dietetics from the University of California, Berkeley, and a master's degree in bio-chemistry from the University of Southern California School of Medicine, Davis did make some serious errors in judgment. For example, Davis rec-ommended raw milk and liquid potassium supplements for infants with colic. These and other unfounded recommendations resulted in numerous cases of harm and at least one death.

Horace Fletcher chewed his way to fame and fortune. Fletcher insisted that food be chewed until almost liquid—thirty to seventy chomps per mouthful.

Carlton Fredricks liked to call himself "America's Foremost Nutritionist." That's pretty impressive for someone with no nutrition or science training. In 1945 Fredricks pled guilty to practicing medicine without a license and then promptly restarted his "medical" practice. In his last years he per-formed nutrition consults from the offices of diet guru Dr. Robert Atkins.

Sylvester Graham's legacy is the graham cracker. This 1820s minister blamed refined flour for most common diseases of his day. Today's graham cracker bears little resemblance to the whole-grain brown bread he pro-moted. He also preached against meat because he believed it inflamed bad tempers and led to sexual excess.

John Harvey Kellogg was the first person to earn over $1 million from health food sales—and that was over 100 years ago. Kellogg was hired by the Seventh Day Adventist Church to run a health sanitarium in Battle Creek, Michigan. Patients were fed handfuls of sterilized bran to promote elimination after every meal. Later John's brother William started the Kel-logg Toasted Corn Flake Company.

Earl Mindell is the king of vitamin supplements. This Ph.D. pharmacist is everywhere, recommending supplements for everyone. And why not? With each new book he writes, a complete line of supplements and related products debuts at the same time: anti-aging supplements with his anti-aging book, soy supplements with his soy book, and so on. Mindell has hooked up with FreeLife International, a pyramid-style, personal selling outfit, to market his wares.

Linus Pauling earned his Nobel prizes for chemistry and peace—not nutrition. He claimed that large amounts of vitamin C could cure or prevent the common cold. Pauling himself took 12,000 mg of vitamin C daily and then upped it to 40,000 mg if he felt a cold coming on. Numerous well-designed, double-blind clinical studies have never been able to duplicate his results. Huge doses of vitamin C act similarly to antihistamines. These drugs work to stop runny noses and watery eyes. Lots of vitamin C, like any over-the-counter antihistamine (Contac, Dristan, Nyquil) can reduce your cold symptoms, but you're still sick.

Charles Post visited Kellogg's sanitarium and saw a business opportunity. He created a competing company and began producing Post Toasted Corn Flakes, Postum, and Grape Nuts, which he promoted as cures for appendicitis, malaria, and consumption. Post surpassed Kellogg and earned $1 million from his products in just one year—1901.

Lendon Smith thought he had the dietary solution for many of his pediatric patients with allergies, hyperactivity, insomnia, and a host of other ailments—avoid white sugar, white flour, pasteurized milk, and then take a variety of supplements to get what you're missing. Smith was first placed on medical probation and then permanently surrendered his medical license rather than face charges of fraud in 1987.

Web Fraud

"Operation Cure-all" is a new law enforcement and consumer education campaign that focuses on stopping Internet quacks and bogus claims for products and treatments touted as cures for various diseases. In 1997 and 1998 the Federal Trade Commission (FTC) surfed the Web and found approximately 800 health-related sites and numerous Internet user groups that contained questionable promotions for products or services. These web sites were sent e-mail messages alerting them that their claims require scientific substantiation and that disseminating unsubstantiated claims violates federal law (FTC News Release, June 1999). Only 28 percent of those sites contacted removed the illegal content or closed their sites in response to notification from the FTC. Violators may be given a civil penalty of $11,000. With soaring profits being made in the supplement industry, an $11,000 fine is no real deterrent.

HANDY HOTLINE to the FTC's consumer response center is 1-877-382-4357 to report or find out about Internet health scams.

LINK UP to http://www.ftc.gov for copies of complaints, proposed settlements, and more information from the Federal Trade Commission on how to safely surf the Web for health information.

Why Bogus Therapies Seem to Work

"At least ten kinds of errors and biases can convince intelligent, honest people that cures have been achieved when they have not," says Barry L. Byerstein from the Brain-Behavior Laboratory, Department of Psychology, Simon Fraser University in British Columbia, Canada. That's why anecdotal reports, testimonials, and uncontrolled observations often inappropriately conclude that some questionable therapies work. Here are the top ten ways fake cures seem to work:

1. The disease may have run its natural course. Your body's own curative powers often work to restore health without any treatment at all.

2. Many diseases are cyclical. Symptoms of chronic conditions such as arthritis, allergies, and stomach complaints often vary dramatically over time. If you try a treatment at a peak time of discomfort, an improvement may just be a normal change in severity.

3. Spontaneous remissions, though quite rare, do happen for both fatal and chronic diseases.

4. The placebo effect. Through a combination of suggestion, belief, or expectancy people do report positive improvement when given a placebo or dummy remedy.

5. Some allegedly cured symptoms are psychosomatic (just in your mind) to begin with.

6. The symptoms of your problem go away and you think you're cured—but the disease is still there.

7. Many people hedge their bets and try lots of therapies at the same time.

8. Sometimes you get misdiagnosed—you never really had what they said you did.

9. By-product benefits produce results that lead to improvement. You try a fad diet that is so low in calories you lose weight and your arthritis improves. It's the weight loss, not the diet, that helped.

10. Some people are mentally ill and can't tell reality from make-believe.

Source: Adapted from Barry L. Beyerstein, *The Skeptical Inquirer,* September/October 1997

LINK UP to http://www.quackwatch.com for an amusing and insightful review operated by Stephen Barrett, M.D., of hundreds of medical quacks and their bogus products and services.

If You Can't Beat 'Em—Join 'Em

Ever wonder what it would be like to be part of a scientific research trial? Now, if you have Internet access, you can log onto a survey and become part of scientific history. This type of survey is self-selected and not randomized, and does have limitations, but you may learn ways to improve your health and nutrition habits. You will certainly gain valuable insight into how study data are collected and all the potential errors that can occur.

LINK UP to http://www.healthsurvey.org to participate in the University of California at Berkeley National Health Study.

Appendices

Glossary: A Mouthful of Nutrition Diction

It takes a whole new language to talk about nutrition today. Here's a collection of new nutrition terms, with pronunciations for those hard-to-say words.

acidophilus (as-uh-DAF-uh-les)   a type of beneficial lactobacillus bacteria that lives in your digestive tract. Imagine a lush, tropical rain forest teeming with life. It's a warm, wet environment where things grow wild. That's what your intestines are like, too. Acidophilus is a **probiotic** that helps keep the healthy bacteria in your gut alive.

antioxidants (an-tea-OX-i-dants)   chemicals that help protect the body from harmful substances called "**free radicals.**" There are two different types of antioxidants in the body: antioxidant enzymes, which prevent too many free radicals from being produced, and dietary antioxidants, which neutralize free radicals and single oxygen cells. You find antioxidants in foods that are rich in vitamins E, C, and selenium.

   To better understand these interactions, imagine yourself at a "couple's only" party. You and your partner are having a great time, as are all the other couples there. You mingle with the other guests, but everyone is in a long-term, committed relationship. Without warning, a wildly charged brute enters the room. He's a free radical and he's all alone. His mission is to break up one of the couples and steal a partner for himself. The free radical bounces from couple to couple trying to find a weak link. He won't give up until he's grabbed himself a mate. Altered by the commotion, a bouncer named antioxidant steps in. Swiftly our antioxidant hero nabs the free radical and escorts him away from the others. Neutralized by the antioxidant, the free radical can't cause any damage. For him, the party's over.

biosource   labeling foods by the geographic area in which they are grown.

biotechnology   the use of advanced scientific techniques to alter and ideally improve selected characteristics of animals and plants.

carcinogen (kar-SIN-oh-gin) anything that can potentially cause cancer. In 1958, Congressman James Delaney from New York introduced legislation to ban carcinogens in the food supply. Distraught over his wife's recent death from cancer, Delaney's proposal said that if any substance is determined to cause cancer in any animal (or human) in any amount, it can't be added to a food. Today's sophisticated technology is capable of finding such minute quantities of these substances that almost all foods could be considered carcinogenic. This was not the case when the Delaney rule was passed. Regardless, the rule is still in effect today.

carotenoid (ka-ROT-in-oid) pigment substances in plants that often form vitamin A. Beta-carotene is the most active form.

chemopreventive agents (keem-o-pre-VEN-tive) parts of food that have the potential to prevent or inhibit cancer.

flavonoids (FLAY-vuh-noyds) originally called vitamin P factors, flavonoids work both inside and outside your cells to protect blood vessels and connective tissue. Flavonoids bring zest to foods in the form of color and flavor. These **phytochemicals** tend to hide in difficult places, like the pith of an orange or the inside of an apple peel. Other good sources of flavonoids include berries, broccoli, celery, cranberries, citrus peel and pulp, grapes and grape juice, green tea, and red wine.

free radicals unstable oxygen molecules that cause problems in the body. In healthy molecules, each atom contains a pair of electrons. While your body works, some of the oxygen molecules lose one of these electrons. When this happens, the formerly stable oxygen molecules become harmful free radicals. These free radicals try to stabilize themselves by taking an electron from another healthy molecule. Some experts estimate that your body is attacked up to ten thousand times a day by free radicals. Free radicals don't usually start a disease process, but they encourage speedy progression of any damage already present. *See also* **antioxidants.**

functional foods those foods that offer a health benefit beyond their vitamin and mineral content, such as antioxidant flavonoids in fruits and vegetables.

isothiocyanates (i-so-thi-o-SI-uh-nates) plant chemicals that may strengthen your body's natural defenses against cancer.

lactobaccillus (LACK-toe-bah-sill-us) a specific strain of beneficial bacteria that lives in your small and lower intestines.

lutein (lew-TEEN) a **carotenoid** found in foods that are dark green and deep orange, plus tomatoes and red peppers. This **phytochemical** helps protect the macula (center portion) of your eyes from oxidation, which results in macular degeneration.

lycopene (LYE-ko-peen)   a colorful red pigment found in foods that may reduce the risk of certain cancers. Tomatoes, watermelon, pink grapefruit, and berries are the best sources of lycopene. Cooking actually enhances their ability to work.

nutraceutical (new-tra-SOO-teh-kal)   a food or food ingredient designed or marketed to provide particular health benefits, including the prevention and treatment of disease. These foods are sometimes called **functional foods** or designer foods. Calcium-fortified orange juice and carrots (when their beta-carotene content is highlighted) would be examples of nutraceuticals.

olestra (Olean)   a no-calorie fat replacer made with sugar and vegetable oil. Olestra has extra molecules that makes it too large to be digested or absorbed, which is why it contains no fat or calories. Since olestra is a fat, it attracts fat-soluble vitamins A, D, E, and K and prevents their absorption in your body. A 1-ounce bag of potato chips made with Olean contains 0 grams of fat and about 70 calories, compared to 10 grams of fat and 150 calories for a 1-ounce bag of full-fat potato chips.

omega-3 (oh-MAY-ga)   a highly unsaturated family of fatty acids often referred to as linolenic acid. They are mostly found in fish and other marine plants and animals (cold water species have the highest concentrations); they are also found in canola oil, flaxseed, leafy green vegetables, and walnuts. Omega-3 is thought to lower "bad" cholesterol and raise "good" cholesterol levels in the blood and may ease some symptoms of rheumatoid arthritis.

omega-6   fats most commonly found in polyunsaturated oils like corn, safflower, soybean, and sunflower. Only in the last hundred years have these oils been commonly eaten. Some estimates suggest that omega-6 fats now make up 90 percent of the polyunsaturated fats in a typical diet. Because we eat most of our unsaturated fats as omega-6 or linolenic fatty acids, we probably don't consume enough omega-3. Try to reduce your consumption of polyunsaturated fats. If you have to substitute another fat, choose a monounsaturated variety like olive or canola oil.

phytochemicals (fi-toe-KEM-eh-kals)   unique plant chemicals from fruits and vegetables that may be essential in boosting health and preventing diseases. They're not vitamins or minerals. So far over four thousand phytochemicals have been identified. It's estimated that only fifty or sixty remain active enough after eating to provide benefits and include lycopene, leutin, and zeaxanthin.

phytoestrogens (fi-toe-ESS-trow-gins) plant chemicals that generate effects similar to the female hormone estrogen. Soy foods, yams, and some legumes are rich in phytoestrogens.

polyphenols (paul-ee-FEE-nalls) compounds that slow anticarcinogenic, antioxidant, antibacterial, and antiviral activity. They can also combine with iron and decrease iron absorption. Green, black, and oolong teas may offer health benefits because they contain **antioxidant** polyphenols.

prebiotics (pree-bye-OT-icks) substances in food that are not digestible by humans, but are digestible by beneficial bacteria that reside in your body.

probiotics (pro-bye-OT-icks) live bacterial supplements used to support beneficial bacteria in the digestive tract.

quercetin (QUER-sa-tin) one of the most powerful **antioxidants.** It acts like a Teflon coating in your bloodstream to prevent the deposit and buildup of sticky cholesterol plaque. Red grapes are a good food source of this antioxidant.

reductive enzymes toxic, cancer-causing by-products of harmful bacteria.

tyramine (TYE-ra-meen) an ingredient in some foods that increases a hormone release that, in turn, causes blood vessels to constrict or tighten. The rebound effect that happens when the blood vessels open wide is throbbing head pain. Foods that contain tyramine include chocolate, aged cheese, and red wine.

Xenical (ZEN-ah-cal) known chemically as orlistat (OR-la-stat), an antifat pill that works by blocking absorption of about one-third of the fat you eat. Due to its blocking function, Xenical can cause unpleasant and embarrassing side effects including gas, oily or loose stools, oily spotting from the rectum, increased urgency to move your bowels, and intestinal cramping. Xenical can also decrease the amount of vitamins A, D, E, and K you absorb from foods.

zeaxanthin (zee-ah-ZAN-thin) a carotenoid found in eggs, dark green leafy vegetables, and corn. This antioxidant has been shown to protect against age-related macular degeneration.

zoochemicals (zoo-KEM-eh-kals) substances in animal foods that help prevent disease.

Ingredient Lists:
What Am I Eating?

Ingredient lists are required on most food products sold. Food components must be listed in order by weight from the most to the least. However, individual variations of the same type of food do not have to be lumped together. For example: honey, sugar, and corn syrup can all be used in a product. Because they are listed separately, total sweeteners are much farther down on the ingredient list than if they were combined.

Lots of unusual-sounding ingredients show up on food labels. Some of the ingredients listed sound like they came from a chemical factory instead of a food plant. But they're not all as bad as they appear. Ascorbic acid may sound like it would eat away at the lining of your stomach. Actually, it's vitamin C. Of the nearly three thousand direct food additives used today, sugar, salt, corn syrup, and dextrose account for more than 90 percent of the total weight. Other common additives include modified starch, yellow mustard, sodium bicarbonate (baking soda), yeast, caramel color, citric acid, carbon dioxide, and black pepper.

Can you guess which foods these ingredient lists describe?

1. Water, starches, cellulose, pectin, fructose, sucrose, glucose, malic acid, citric acid, succinic acid, anisyl propionate, amyl acetate, ascorbic acid, beta-carotene, riboflavin, thiamin, niacin, phosphorus, potassium.

2. Water, triglycerides of stearic, palmitic, oleic and linoleic acids, myosin, actin, glycogen, collagen, lecithin, cholesterol, dipotassium phosphate, myoglobin, urea.

You guessed correctly if you answered cantaloupe for the first and steak for the second.

Labeling Lingo: What's Reduced, Low, and Free

Many people get confused about what is on the food label and the subtle differences among what is reduced, low, or even free. There are simple definitions for the terms on a food label for specific nutrients and the health claims stated.

If the label says:	One serving can have no more than:
Calorie free	5 calories
Low calorie	40 calories
Sugar free	½ gm sugar
Fat free	½ gm fat
Low fat	3 gm fat
Sodium free	5 mg sodium
Low sodium	140 mg sodium
Cholesterol free	2 mg cholesterol and 2 gm saturated fat
Low cholesterol	20 mg cholesterol and 2 gm saturated fat
Reduced	25% less of that ingredient than the standard version of the product
Lean (meat products only)	10 g total fat and 4 g saturated fat and 95 mg cholesterol
Extra lean (meat products only)	5 g total fat and 2 g saturated fat and 95 mg cholesterol

Source: FDA Regulations, 1993, 1994, and USDA Regulations, 1994

There are other familiar words on the label that may not mean what you think they do. Here are some, with their technical definitions:

Enriched: The vitamins thiamin, riboflavin, and niacin and the mineral iron have been added at varying levels to the product to replace what's lost during processing.

Fortified: Vitamins and/or minerals have been added to a product in amounts higher than 10 percent of what's normally found in that food.

Healthy: The FDA is proposing a definition of "healthy." The term would be applicable to foods that are low in fat and saturated fat and that do not contain more than 480 mg of sodium or 60 mg of cholesterol per serving.

Light or Lite: These words can mean one of three things:

1. In reference to fat or calories, a food can be altered to contain one-third fewer calories or 50 percent less fat than the regular version of that product.

2. A 50 percent reduction from the amount of sodium in the regular product is required.

3. The term "light" can also be used to describe the color and texture of a food. "Light" pancakes may just be fluffy, not low fat or low calorie. When light is used this way, it must tell you which attribute the food is light in.

Good source: One serving contains 10 to 19 percent of the Daily Value for a particular nutrient.

High or Excellent Source: One serving contains 20 percent or more of the Daily Value for a particular nutrient.

Organic: At the time this book was printed, there was no final ruling on national organic standards.

The FDA also allows a list of nutrient-disease relationships on food labels such as:

- Calcium and osteoporosis
- Fat and cancer
- Saturated fat and cholesterol and heart disease
- Fiber-containing fruits, vegetables, and grain products and cancer
- Fiber-containing fruits, vegetables, and grain products and heart disease
- Sodium and hypertension
- Fruits and vegetables, and cancer
- Whole-grain foods and heart disease
- Whole-grain foods and cancer
- Soy and heart disease

Federal Nutrients Standards

DAILY VALUES (USED ON FOOD LABELS)

Daily Reference Values (DRVs)[a]

Food Component	DRV
fat	65 g[b]
saturated fatty acids	20 g
cholesterol	300 mg[c]
total carbohydrate	300 g
fiber	25 g
sodium	2,400 mg
potassium	3,500 mg
protein[d]	50 g

[a] Based on 2,000 calories a day for adults and children over 4 only.
[b] (g) grams
[c] (mg) milligrams
[d] DRV for protein does not apply to certain populations; Reference Daily Intake (RDI) for protein has been established for these groups: children 1 to 4 years: 16 g; infants under 1 year: 14 g; pregnant women: 60 g; nursing mothers: 65 g.

Reference Daily Intakes (RDIs)[a]

Nutrient	Amount	Nutrient	Amount
vitamin A	5,000 International Units (IU)	folic acid	0.4 mg
vitamin C	60 mg	vitamin B_{12}	6 µg[b]
thiamin	1.5 mg	phosphorus	1.0 g
riboflavin	1.7 mg	iodine	150 µg
niacin	20 mg	magnesium	400 mg
calcium	1.0 g	zinc	15 mg
iron	18 mg	copper	2 mg
vitamin D	400 IU	biotin	0.3 mg
vitamin E	30 IU	panthothenic acid	10 mg
vitamin B_6	2.0 mg		

[a] Formerly the U.S. RDA, based on National Academy of Sciences' 1968 Recommended Dietary Allowances.
[b] (µg) micrograms

Source: R. Kurtzweil, "'Daily Values' Encourage Healthy Diet," *FDA Consumer*, May 1993, pp. 40–45

Dietary Reference Intakes: Recommended Levels for Individual Intake[a]

Life-stage group	Calcium (mg/d)	Phosporus (mg/d)	Magnesium (mg/d)	Vitamin D[bc] (µg/d)	Fluoride (mg/d)	Thiamin (mg/d)	Riboflavin (mg/d)	Niacin[d] (mg/d)	Vitamin B$_6$ (mg/d)	Folate[e] (µg/d)	Vitamin B$_{12}$ (µg/d)	Pantothenic Acid (mg/d)	Biotin (µg/d)	Choline[f] (mg/d)
Infants														
0–6 mo	210*	100*	30*	5*	0.01*	0.2*	0.3*	2*	0.1*	65*	0.4*	1.7*	5*	125*
7–12 mo	270*	275*	75*	5*	0.5*	0.3*	0.4*	4*	0.3*	80*	0.5*	1.8*	6*	150*
Children														
1–3 y	500*	460	80	5*	0.7*	0.5	0.5	6	0.5	150	0.9	2*	8*	200*
4–8 y	800*	500	130	5*	1*	0.6	0.6	8	0.6	200	1.2	3*	12*	250*
Males														
9–13 y	1,300*	1,250	240	5*	2*	0.9	0.9	12	1.0	300	1.8	4*	20*	375*
14–18 y	1,300*	1,250	410	5*	3*	1.2	1.3	16	1.3	400	2.4	5*	25*	550*
19–30 y	1,000*	700	400	5*	4*	1.2	1.3	16	1.3	400	2.4	5*	30*	550*
31–50 y	1,000*	700	420	5*	4*	1.2	1.3	16	1.3	400	2.4	5*	30*	550*
51–70 y	1,200*	700	420	10*	4*	1.2	1.3	16	1.7	400	2.4[g]	5*	30*	550*
>70 y	1,200*	700	420	15*	4*	1.2	1.3	16	1.7	400	2.4[g]	5*	30*	550*
Females														
9–13 y	1,300*	1,250	240	5*	2*	0.9	0.9	12	1.0	300	1.8	4*	20*	375*
14–18 y	1,300*	1,250	360	5*	3*	1.0	1.0	14	1.2	400[h]	2.4	5*	25*	400*
19–30 y	1,000*	700	310	5*	3*	1.1	1.1	14	1.3	400[h]	2.4	5*	30*	425*
31–50 y	1,000*	700	320	5*	3*	1.1	1.1	14	1.3	400[h]	2.4	5*	30*	425*
51–70 y	1,200*	700	320	10*	3*	1.1	1.1	14	1.5	400	2.4[g]	5*	30*	425*
>70 y	1,200*	700	320	15*	3*	1.1	1.1	14	1.5	400	2.4[g]	5*	30*	425*
Pregnancy														
≤18 y	1,300*	1,250	400	5*	3*	1.4	1.4	18	1.9	600[i]	2.6	6*	30*	450*
19–30 y	1,000*	700	350	5*	3*	1.4	1.4	18	1.9	600[i]	2.6	6*	30*	450*
31–50 y	1,000*	700	360	5*	3*	1.4	1.4	18	1.9	600[i]	2.6	6*	30*	450*
Lactation														
≤18 y	1,300*	1,250	360	5*	3*	1.5	1.6	17	2.0	500	2.8	7*	35*	550*
19–30 y	1,000*	700	310	5*	3*	1.5	1.6	17	2.0	500	2.8	7*	35*	550*
31–50 y	1,000*	700	320	5*	3*	1.5	1.6	17	2.0	500	2.8	7*	35*	550*

Tolerable Upper Intake Levels[a] (ULs) for Certain Nutrients

Life-stage group	Calcium (g/d)	Phosporus (g/d)	Magnesium[b] (mg/d)	Vitamin D (µg/d)	Fluoride (mg/d)	Niacin[c] (mg/d)	Vitamin B6 (mg/d)	Synthetic folic acid (µg/d)[c]	Choline (g/d)
0–6 mo	ND[d]	ND	ND	25	0.7	ND	ND	ND	ND
7–12 mo	ND	ND	ND	25	0.9	ND	ND	ND	ND
1–3 y	2.5	3	65	50	1.3	10	30	300	1.0
4–8 y	2.5	3	110	50	2.2	15	40	400	1.0
9–13 y	2.5	4	350	50	10	20	60	600	2.0
14–18 y	2.5	4	350	50	10	30	80	800	3.0
19–70 y	2.5	4	350	50	10	35	100	1,000	3.5
>70 y	2.5	3	350	50	10	35	100	1,000	3.5
Pregnancy									
≤18 y	2.5	3.5	350	50	10	30	80	800	3.0
19–50 y	2.5	3.5	350	50	10	35	100	1,000	3.5
Lactation									
≤18 y	2.5	4	350	50	10	30	80	800	3.0
19–50 y	2.5	4	350	50	10	35	100	1,000	3.5

[a]UL = the maximum level of daily nutrient intake that is likely to pose no risk of adverse effects. Unless otherwise specified, the UL represents total intake from food, water, and supplements. Due to lack of suitable data, ULs could not be established for thiamin, riboflavin, vitamin B₁₂, pantothenic acid, or biotin. In the absence of ULs, extra caution may be warranted in consuming levels above recommended intakes.

[b]The UL for magnesium represents intake from a pharmacological agent only and does not include intake from food and water.

[c]The ULs for niacin and synthetic folic acid apply to forms obtained from supplements, fortified foods, or a combination of the two.

[d]ND: Not determinable due to lack of data of adverse effects in this age group and concern with regard to lack of ability to handle excess amounts. Source of intake should be from food only to prevent high levels of intake.

Food and Nutrition Board, National Academy of Sciences—National Research Council

Recommended Dietary Allowances,[a] Revised 1989

Designed for the maintenance of good nutrition of practically all healthy people in the United States

Category	Age (years) or Condition	Weight[b] (kg)	Weight[b] (lb)	Height[b] (cm)	Height[b] (in)	Protein (g)	Fat-Soluble Vitamins — Vitamin A (µg RE)[c]	Vitamin D (µg)[d]	Vitamin E (mg α-TE)[e]	Vitamin K (µg)	Water-Soluble Vitamins — Vitamin C (mg)	Thiamin (mg)	Riboflavin (mg)	Niacin (µg NE)[f]	Vitamin B6 (mg)	Folate (µg)	Vitamin B12 (µg)	Minerals — Calcium (mg)	Phosphorus (mg)	Magnesium (µg)	Iron (mg)	Zinc (mg)	Iodine (µg)	Selenium (µg)
Infants	0.0–0.5	6	13	60	24	13	375	7.5	3	5	30	0.3	0.4	5	0.3	25	0.3	400	300	40	6	5	40	10
	0.5–1.0	9	20	71	28	14	375	10	4	10	35	0.4	0.5	6	0.6	35	0.5	600	500	60	10	5	50	15
Children	1–3	13	29	90	35	16	400	10	6	15	40	0.7	0.8	9	1.0	50	0.7	800	800	80	10	10	70	20
	4–6	20	44	112	44	24	500	10	7	20	45	0.9	1.1	12	1.1	75	1.0	800	800	120	10	10	90	20
	7–10	28	62	132	52	28	700	10	7	30	45	1.0	1.2	13	1.4	100	1.4	800	800	170	10	10	120	30
Males	11–14	45	99	157	62	45	1,000	10	10	45	50	1.3	1.5	17	1.7	150	2.0	1,200	1,200	270	12	15	150	40
	15–18	66	145	176	69	59	1,000	10	10	65	60	1.5	1.8	20	2.0	200	2.0	1,200	1,200	400	12	15	150	50
	19–24	72	160	177	70	58	1,000	10	10	70	60	1.5	1.7	19	2.0	200	2.0	1,200	1,200	350	10	15	150	70
	25–50	79	174	176	70	63	1,000	5	10	80	60	1.5	1.7	19	2.0	200	2.0	800	800	350	10	15	150	70
	51+	77	170	173	68	63	1,000	5	10	80	60	1.2	1.4	15	2.0	200	2.0	800	800	350	10	15	150	70
Females	11–14	46	101	157	62	46	800	10	8	45	50	1.1	1.3	15	1.4	150	2.0	1,200	1,200	280	15	12	150	45
	15–18	55	120	163	64	44	800	10	8	55	60	1.1	1.3	15	1.5	180	2.0	1,200	1,200	300	15	12	150	50
	19–24	58	128	164	65	46	800	10	8	60	60	1.1	1.3	15	1.6	180	2.0	1,200	1,200	280	15	12	150	55
	25–50	63	138	163	64	50	800	5	8	65	60	1.1	1.3	15	1.6	180	2.0	800	800	280	15	12	150	55
	51+	65	143	160	63	50	800	5	8	65	60	1.0	1.2	13	1.6	180	2.0	800	800	280	10	12	150	55
Pregnant						60	800	10	10	65	70	1.5	1.6	17	2.2	400	2.2	1,200	1,200	320	30	15	175	65
Lactating	1st 6 months					65	1,300	12	12	65	95	1.6	1.8	20	2.1	280	2.6	1,200	1,200	355	15	19	200	75
	2nd 6 months					62	1,200	11	11	65	90	1.6	1.7	20	2.1	260	2.6	1,200	1,200	340	15	16	200	75

[a] The allowances, expressed as average daily intakes over time, are intended to provide for individual variations among the most normal persons as they live in the United States under usual environmental stresses. Diets should be based on a variety of common foods in order to provide other nutrients for which human requirements have been less well defined.

[b] Weights and heights of Reference Adults are actual medians for the U.S. population of the designated age, as reported by NHANES II. The use of these figures does not imply that the height-to-weight rations are ideal.

[c] Retinol equivalents. 1 retinol equivalent = 1 µg retinol or 6 µg β-carotene.

[d] As cholecalciferol. 10 µg cholecalciferol = 400 IU of vitamin D.

[e] α-Tocopherol equivalents. 1 mg d-α tocopherol = 1 α-TE.

[f] 1 NE (niacin equivalent) is equal to 1 mg of niacin or 60 mg of dietary tryptophan.

Index